Socks

And

Stuff

By

Lynne Mattick

DEDICATION

This book is dedicated to Jo and Rachel, my beautiful daughters and Neil, the Brother from the North, who has supported me through everything.

CONTENTS

Socks and Stuff

Chapter One

Advice to struggling new writers – always start with something gripping that will make the reader want to read on. So where shall I start? With my socks!

Those socks had started some sort of teenage rebellion and were flatly refusing to behave as I wished. They were twins and although identical in appearance, they were not identical in character. One of them always emerged from the washing machine the right way out, swung neatly on the line and lay quietly in the drawer where I laid it. The other never seemed to be in the dark wash (unless hidden halfway up a trouser leg) but was always wrapped round a pair of pale pink ballet tights, seemingly attempting to strangle them. Thus the ballet tights are heading towards grey rather than pink and the sock is gaining in power every wash day. The toe of the said sock is usually trying to reach the ribbed top from the inside and if I ever get it as far as the line, it swings vigorously to and fro until it manages to wrap itself round the line, snagging two or three pegs in the process. Deep within the drawer, it struggles to escape from its more amenable partner and once having done so, it burrows deeper and deeper until it finds a rarely used pair of tights and proceeds to play hide and seek. It is only when I have emptied the drawer and have spread the contents over my bed that the sock turns up, smiling in a mysterious way and claiming that it was in the right place all along. All I had to do was look more carefully.

By now, I am usually late, so the underwear remains spread across the bed until I am about to collapse into it at the end of the day. (The bed that is, not the underwear). Goodness knows what the poor window cleaner must think as he stares through the glass (only possible AFTER he has cleaned it) at the tangled heap of unmatching socks, large knickers, twisted tights, pretty lace handkerchiefs and a lacy suspender belt from days that are so long ago that they cannot be lightly brought to mind. However, it remains there because one day, I may just get into it again.... this despite the fact that I am allergic to lace and never even wore the thing.

Anyway, to return to this particular Monday, I was seated on the bottom stair attempting to put on my socks. Something was definitely wrong! I had managed to prop my left foot on my right knee and could just touch the sock with my toes but seemed unable to get any further. By dint of a little hooking movement, I finally pushed my toes into the reluctant sock and gradually eased it over my foot. From there it was easy. All I needed to do was to crouch on the hall floor with one leg stretched elegantly behind me and the other bent double under me and I could pull the sock up to its proper length.

I returned to my original position on the stairs and eyed the remaining sock somewhat nervously. I really wanted to go out today. It was bright and sunny and I had promised myself a slow stroll to the post box – my first outing alone for a couple of weeks. The prospect hung before me like a tantalising gem, sparkling with excitement and not a little danger. But first I had to put on my other sock.

I was unable to place my right foot on my left knee so I lay across the stair with the leg bent behind me but the sock just shrugged its ribbed shoulders and hung dangling from my outstretched fingers. I changed tactics then and tried to take it by surprise by reversing my leg position. I picked myself up off the floor, rescued the sock from its new position under the doormat and considered my options. I shouted at the sock and it just turned away in dumb defiance. I pleaded with it and it slipped to the floor, disgusted at my humiliating performance. By now, my back was aching, the muscles in my chest wall were complaining and my numb left arm had had enough and had gone on strike, refusing to raise itself higher than waist level. There was only one thing left to do and so I did it. I gave up. I hurled the rebellious sock across the hall where it lay smirking on the edge of the radiator before sliding down behind it to join the two pairs of pants, a tea towel and a vocabulary book (left to dry after an incident with milk) which had lived down there for some time avoiding all capture. In desperate need of a quiet sit down with coffee, I walked with one sock on and one sock off, into the kitchen. A few minutes later, I was comfortably ensconced in the chair with a cup of hot coffee, a biscuit (was that really necessary?) and my "Patients' Guide to Mastectomy". I thumbed through the index but could find no reference to socks anywhere. There was a great deal about discomfort, numbness, lymphodoema, scar tissue and psychological problems but no mention of socks. They never mention socks in cancer leaflets and it's about time someone did. I would mention it at my next visit to the Hospital.

Meanwhile, I still had a pile of thank you letters to post, one sock on and nothing to do but think.

Chapter Two

Some four years ago, a young and eager cell had held a meeting low down in my left breast. He had finally had enough of being squashed and pummelled for many years and yet receiving no recognition. He wanted out! He gathered a group of like-minded cells and set off on his path to freedom.

"What do we want?" He would shout.

"Freedom!" came the response.

"How do we get it?"

"Er.. we're not sure exactly…"

"By fizzing!" Yelled the enthusiastic Young Leader.

"Fizzing? OK if you say so," agreed his mates and so they fizzed.

This was an uncomfortable and slightly worrying sensation for me who had spent the last years fully expecting a recurrence of the cancer first diagnosed and treated in 1985. However, the doctors at the Hospital could do no more than tell me to keep an eye on things and come back in a year again.

After a year, the Young Leader sought advice from older and wiser cells. Some recommended that he enlarged his support group and got backing from other cells. Others said that it just wasn't worth it. He should go back to his day job and forget about freedom. These were the old thickened cells on the fringes of previous scar tissue and the Young Leader considered them to be unnecessarily cynical. He ignored them and increased his group of supporters, redoubling his efforts to attract attention to himself.

Would it work? He awaited the annual mammogram with mounting excitement.

In spite of the fact that I have these annual mammograms, I never fail to be amazed at how flat the average breast can become under pressure. This occasion was no exception. I left my friend ensconced in the waiting room with an elderly and tattered copy of Hello! Magazine and entered the tiny cubicle where I would remove my 'upper garments' as instructed. Then, shivering and feeling a little vulnerable, I stood in the middle of the room whilst my name, date of birth and serial number were checked. The machine loomed large in the corner of the room and I approached with my usual mixed feelings. This would be at best uncomfortable but was a form of security for me. If changes had occurred, this machine would probably find them.

Picture the scene. My left hand was clinging to a large plastic handle above and forward of my head level. My right arm embraced the machine as far as I could possibly reach. My left, C-cup breast was sandwiched between two thick plates of Perspex. My right, E-cup breast was seeking to join its companion by insinuating itself under the Perspex layer. This pinched and so the breast was manhandled (or woman-handled) out of the way and sort of tucked under my outstretched arm. At this point, my rather impressive stomach decided that it was feeling left out of things and made a break to join my left breast. This, too, was pushed aside without ceremony and my upper body now became on very intimate terms with the machine whilst my lower body maintained a rather frigid and disapproving attitude. My bottom protruded into the room and my stomach was sucked in as hard as possible (no mean feat when you are well over 15 stone in weight, most of it centred on the said stomach!)

The two plates were now drawn inexorably together and the C-cup took on the distinct appearance of a rather ill-made pancake. Since this is the side that had already suffered the indignities of surgery and radiotherapy, the whole operation was not without pain but it was at this point that the kindly acolyte to the machine said brightly, "Comfortable? Then just hold that position and your breath."

She disappeared behind a screen, pressed buttons and after a brief whirring sound, advised me that I could release my breath just as the machine loosed its grip on my pancake which miraculously sprang back into its original, sagging condition. The whole procedure was then repeated on the other side and the E-cup sniggered and made comments about the difference between spectacular crepes and drop-scones while my stomach sulked and dreamed of flatter days.

I was finally decanted back into the waiting room while the pictures were checked. Several pages of Hello! later, the acolyte reappeared and informed me that there was a problem with the machine and I would have to have another picture taken of one side. The Young Leader deep inside C-cup held his breath. Had it worked or was this really just a machine malfunction. After so many mammograms, we both knew the procedure and that this comment was sometimes (though not always) a euphemism to cover the discovery of mysterious and unexplained changes.

The whole procedure was duly repeated and I was sent off to consume much needed coffee and chocolate and then to return home to pass a nail-biting couple of weeks before my next clinic appointment.

The Young Leader held a meeting to celebrate but little did he know that on the other side of the breast, a rival faction was quietly and systematically gathering strength.

Chapter Three

The date for my clinic appointment duly arrived and I was examined by a rather nice young doctor with very soft hands. He then informed me that the mammo had shown up something suspicious and that he would like me to have an ultrasound scan to investigate further.

This meant making yet another appointment and another two week wait. But time soon passes and I made my way down long empty corridors full of abandoned paint pots and dust sheets to the ultrasound department which was in the process of being repainted. Incarcerated in a tiny cell-like cubicle, I somehow managed to remove my jumper and bra without actually bruising my arms on the walls and entered the darkened room beyond. The man who wielded the scanner and ruled this humming domain, was a kindly looking person with a sense of humour and a gentle nature that hid his awful secret. I lay on the bed, tipped at forty five degrees, smothered with a somewhat cool gel and submitted to the roving scanner. The kindly-looking face revealed its true nature. A puzzled and anxious frown began to creep across the forehead. It seemed a little reluctant and shy at first but soon gathered courage, egged on by the flickering images on the screen. As the scanner moved to the lower slopes of C-cup, the frown drifted upwards towards the hairline in a vain attempt to become a look of pleasant surprise. The hair was having none of it and soon sent the frown packing with a stern admonition to be more truthful. The frown deepened and made a bid for the top of the nose. This was much more successful and as the eyes half closed in order to peer more closely at the screen, the frown made its final assault upon the face and was rewarded with that ultimate accolade.

"I need a second opinion here," said the man and left to find one. The second opinion examined the screen aided by another trainee frown. She even took over control of the scanner which rolled in ever decreasing circles down towards my left armpit.

Deep inside C-cup, chaos reigned. The Young Leader was jumping up and down, trying to draw attention to himself, but he was too far away and could not make his presence felt. On the other side of the hill, the rival faction had disbanded and its various members had returned to their usual daily life. The scanner probed and rolled and the frown and the second opinion gazed from the screen to the mammo report and back again. The frown took his rightful place as master of his domain and nodded slightly at the second opinion. Then came the verdict.

"No, there's nothing there at all. It was probably a cyst brought on by hormonal changes and which then vanished. They do that when you get to a certain age." My fifty years shuddered with humiliation and then reasserted themselves.

"I'm not that old," I protested mildly. The man assured me that I knew what he meant and that he was just glad to be able to give me such good news. The second opinion smiled briefly and returned to her mysterious work on the other side of the screen. The leader of the rival faction sent a message to his scattered supporters to inform them that the strategy had worked and that they had completely fooled the powers that be. The Young Leader hunched his shoulders in bitter disappointment and began to lay his plans for growth and personal development.

Yet another clinic appointment confirmed the results and I was free for another year. Relief was enormous and yet still tempered by a slight uncertainty. I determined to get on with my life but to remain vigilant.

The year passed. My husband of over 22 years departed in search of a different life leaving my little family devastated. My beloved cat died of cancer just after Christmas. Two new cats, a mother and son, joined our family in May. My elder daughter departed for a teaching year in France as part of her degree course. My younger daughter left her primary school and entered the homework strewn life of Secondary School. We gradually learned how to live as a single parent family and life rolled ever onwards until it was October yet again.

I will not repeat the mammogram scenario. A re-reading of chapter two will provide you with exactly the information you need except for the fact that this time, there was no recall for another picture. I headed towards the clinic appointment with no technical basis for anxiety but the Young Leader had not been idle during the year. He had re-grouped and gathered in more supporters including spies from the rival faction group who promised to keep him appraised of any further competition. The nice young doctor had been replaced by another nice young doctor who informed me gently that the mammo had shown up something suspicious and that he would like me to have an ultrasound. It was then that the rival faction's work came to light. We realised that the scan had concentrated on the wrong area last time and I was now rather more than slightly anxious.

The frown was alone in ultrasound – the second opinion had just left armed with a box of slides and tubes. The frown had obviously been practising during the year and had now grown to full maturity. The pleasant smile slipped out for coffee and the frown and the scanner were working in perfect harmony. The second opinion had been replaced by the probing fingers which alternated with the scanner and caused the frown to deepen even more.

Finally, the frown sat back and said, "Well, the scanner isn't really showing anything much." The scanner blushed and hid its glowing head. "But I can definitely feel something there." The fingers cheered silently and added this information to their anti-machine campaign.

"I think I will do a fine needle aspiration just to

make sure. Would you like a local anaesthetic? It can sometimes be worse than the fine-needle." Not convinced by that, I opted for the local anaesthetic which was painless and he placed the scanner just above the Young Leader's vantage point. The fine-needle was inserted into the breast and directed towards the gathered supporters below. Suddenly, the Young Leader froze in a moment of indecision. "Down!" he shouted and his well trained troops obediently threw themselves flat. Would the fine-needle locate the cowering supporters or even the Young Leader himself? Was the game finally up? Fine-needle withdrew looking enigmatic and dressings were placed on the already burgeoning bruise. Only time and yet another clinic appointment would tell, but by now, there was no doubt in my mind at all and I set about putting a stand-by life into action.

Chapter Four

My reasons for this were perfectly logical. I foresaw that an operation would be needed no matter what the outcome of the tests. If the test proved positive, then the only possible plan of action was to undergo an operation. If the test proved negative, then I was sure that they would suggest the operation anyway. Nineteen years previously, all tests had proved negative but I had insisted on a lumpectomy as I was considering a second pregnancy and could not have stood the pain of breastfeeding with my small intruder. The doctors had agreed and we were all somewhat shocked when the tumour turned out to be malignant. Two operations, six weeks' radiotherapy and many years of annual checks later, I was sure that the doctors would want to remove this lump too. The Young Leader was counting on this and eagerly awaited his route to freedom. So I set about re-organising my daily life.

My first problem was to find child care for my younger daughter. She would need someone with whom she could feel at ease and who could be her chauffeur, homework help, alarm clock and shoulder on which to cry if necessary. Answer to prayer came in the form of my Brother from the North. He needed to take a week's holiday before the end of March and he also needed a bolt hole. As the younger daughter's uncle and god-father, he would be perfect and what's more, he would be able to come down with the minimum of notice. My plan was beginning to take shape. I had a huge network of support around me and proceeded to delegate various duties – just in case!

Two weeks later, secure in the knowledge that my plans were all in place and that I would be able to accept any date for an operation, I set off once again for hospital. The offers of physical support had been pouring in and I could have filled a minibus with those who wanted to accompany me. In the end, I chose just two people – the two Js - and we set off, though not in a minibus.

I decided to leave one J in the waiting room as she had already been through two bouts of this herself and I was more than anxious about her in this situation. The other J and I squeezed ourselves into the tiny cubicle and yet again, I removed my upper garments, concealed by a curtain and fought my way into the carefully laundered gown. I pushed back the curtain and heaped my clothes onto J's waiting knees. The Young Leader waited in anticipation and I waited with him. Another doctor entered the room accompanied by a staff nurse and proceeded to examine me. He informed me that the Fine-Needle had made his journey of discovery into C-cup but had found nothing. All was well. A relative of a previously seen Frown now made its way onto the young doctor's face. His probing fingers moved backwards and forwards around the slopes of C-cup and the Frown deepened. The Young Leader shivered. Had he made a mistake after all? Was he following the right course of action? He dispersed his support and decided to lay low. Cowering inside C-cup, he wriggled his way out from underneath the fingers and managed to avoid detection.

The young doctor scratched his head and the Frown changed its tactics and rushed up into the receding hairline to become an expression of astonishment.

"I can feel nothing there," remarked the young doctor. "Can you feel it?" But the Young Leader's hiding place was secure and I could feel nothing either.

"Sit up please," came the innocent request and I was at once plunged into indecision.

Sitting up from a prone position was never easy as I had a back problem. Usually, I rolled over onto my stomach, raised myself on all fours and then was able to twist round into the seated position. I could foresee difficulties if I followed this course of action. Undoubtedly, the loss of any shred of dignity was a major consideration but far outweighing that was the knowledge of simple physics. The bed, upon which I lay half naked, was a very narrow, very high hospital examination couch. If I were to roll so much as an inch, then the laws of gravity would take over and I would be precipitated onto the floor with the resultant loss of dignity and a probable need for a visit to the fracture clinic. Rolling was definitely not an option. I would have to attempt the difficult manoeuvre of sitting up straight from prone. This had its own drawbacks. The young doctor was close by and I feared that I would hit him with my flailing arms. The staff nurse was crammed into the only available space left to her, which was between the sink and the bin for disposable waste and she would not be able to come to my rescue should the need arise. Lastly, my dignity made a brief speech, pleading against this action. J had followed my battles with weight for many years. She knew to the ounce exactly what my scales showed me but she would now be able to see the awful truth. It would no longer be hidden beneath tunics and loose jumpers or be smoothed out by the prone position. My stomach would be revealed in all its glory and I was ashamed and anxious. I could not lie there unmoving for much longer. I considered the pros and cons. There was no alternative. My dignity shuddered in dismay and prepared for humiliation as I struggled up from prone.

"Nothing there!" was the puzzled reaction. "Could you stand up and face me please?"

My dignity had fled the room realising that it was already too cramped in there and that it would be better off elsewhere. I stood obediently and faced him – and thus also faced the staff nurse and the non-flinching J.

"Hands behind your head please." I now felt like a prisoner in a rather low-budget TV show where space was at a premium. I placed my hands behind my head and was subjected to yet more probings. The Frown was back now and I waited for the response from the young doctor.

"Nothing to be felt. Come back in a year."

"No!" I cried out. "That's too long to wait. Can't you just remove it?"

The Young Leader waited for the reply. He was very confused. Did he want to escape or not? His supporters were muttering round him, threatening to abandon him if he did not make some decisions and make them fast.

The young doctor looked at me thoughtfully.

"I will go and ask a doctor." With that he disappeared into the inner sanctum leaving me in a state of extreme anxiety. Was he not a doctor? Was he then the cleaner? The man who refilled the vending machines perhaps? A patient from one of the distant wards where mind and body were treated hand in hand? The staff nurse did not seem concerned by his actions and remained quietly wedged.

Ten long minutes passed and the young doctor reappeared with a new, lower offer.

"Three months?" he suggested persuasively. "It's the best I can offer."

I reviewed my options. My stand-by plan of action was in place now. I had worried and fretted for long enough. I caught J's eye and she nodded encouragingly.

"No. I don't want to wait any more." I said. But the young doctor had lost interest in me. Other, more pliable patients awaited his ministrations and, shrugging, he left me.

I was at a loss now. What more could I do? The staff nurse unwedged herself and spoke in a way that suggested that she understood my situation. She explained that they could not operate if the Young Leader was not to be found as they were not prepared to butcher me just in case there should be something there. She suggested that I might like to see the consultant – the Great Italian. I agreed with haste and she went off to make the appointment for me whilst I struggled back into my clothes, recalled my dignity from its hiding place and went back to the waiting room with J. We found the other J in an obvious state of apprehension as she was apparently reading her book upside down. It was only then that I realised the length of time that I had been in the tiny cubicle and the worry that I had inflicted on her. She has a forgiving nature and we made our way back to the non-minibus, armed with an appointment with the Great Italian for four weeks hence and the realisation that I may just have to alter my stand-by plan of action after all.

Chapter Five

In this world of ours, it is often said that it's not what you know but who you know that counts and that proved to be the case for me. The four week wait to see the Great Italian stretched before me – a time to be filled with anxiety. However, one of my colleagues at the school where I worked stepped into this void. It was Thursday and playtime and we were both on duty. The rain had stopped and the children were channelled out of their rooms, bundled reluctantly into hats, gloves and suitable outerwear and released into the wild. We huddled into our coats as we watched hordes of energetic six year olds swooping around the strategically placed sandpits, playhouses, see-saws and vertically challenged wooden pencils. We distracted the more enthusiastic among them as they vigorously wielded brooms in an attempt to brush away the puddles and consoled those who wept bitterly because their precious stickers had blown away into the biting January wind. In the space of twenty five minutes we were mediators, counsellors, referees, peace envoys and sergeant majors. As we patrolled our terrain with watchful eyes, alternating warm smiles with sad and disappointed frowns, we found the time to chat. During these odd moments the Colleague informed me that she also worked at the Hospital and knew the Great Italian very well. She offered to try to bring forward my appointment by pulling a few strings. I accepted with alacrity and thanked God yet again for all the wonderful people around me.

She managed to shave two weeks off my waiting time and so it was that I was once more ensconced in the tiny cubicle waiting to be prodded like a side of beef.

I had not seen the Great Italian for many years although it was always his clinic I attended. On the last occasion we had met, I had been considering my weight problems (no change there then) and had come to the conclusion that my problem was psychological and nothing to do with eating too much after all. This arose from the fact that at the time of my previous incarceration in this hospital, I had weighed a slim 9stone 12 lbs. This was directly a result of my attendance at a slimming club combined with running four times a week. I distinctly recall the words of the Bone Scanner as she ran her supermarket-type scanner up and down my naked, shivering and water filled body, "It's such a pleasure to do this on someone so slim for a change." I had never heard these words before and treasured them. Radiographers told me to put on weight – about a stone would do – and I lost no time in obeying them. After all, they were white coats and should be obeyed at all times. This is a reaction that I later regretted as the stone was later joined by several other recruits eager to visit this place where they would apparently be accepted willingly. They have never left me.

I associated being slim with having breast cancer – after all, the magazines all put weight loss at the top of their lists of 'things to watch out for'. I conveniently ignored the word 'unexplained' that always came before the 'weight loss' bit. Psychologically, slim equalled cancer and so I protected myself by staying well overweight. The Young Doctor of the time recommended that I talk to the Great Italian and he appeared as if by magic. He listened carefully to everything I had to say and he listened, too, to all that I did not say. Finally, he suggested that I saw a counsellor and I spent several weeks visiting the psychological medicine department. My counsellor helped with many things, but I never got to the bottom of my weight block.

I trusted the Great Italian and waited impatiently for him to enter my tiny cubicle. If **he** told me to wait a year, then I would listen to him and reconsider my options. The Great Italian entered and shook my hand. He listened carefully to what I had to say and pondered my situation. He agreed that he could not operate without further proof and he suggested my next course of action. Deep in the bowels of the hospital, Fine-Needle felt the vibrations of the Great Italian's next words. "I suggest a Large Needle biopsy." Fine-Needle quivered in humiliation and shame. He had failed and now the big guns were entering the field. I thanked the Great Italian and left for the rapid Diagnostic Unit (known as ARDAC) to spend a further hour waiting to make an appointment with Large-Needle. The word 'rapid' seemed to be extremely inappropriate but after much waiting, the appointment was made and I returned home for yet another wait.

Throughout my weeks of test and waitings and tests and results, I had surrounded myself with support from my peers. Apart from the absent Husband and the Brother from the North, they were none of them related to me and whilst I knew they loved me, they were not emotionally bound to me by shared genes or day by day knowledge. However, there still remained a generation each side of mine and they would have to receive the information at some point. At which point exactly was causing me no little concern. My parents could worry for England and I wanted to wait until I had something concrete about which to worry. The fear of what might be is so much worse than what actually is and thus unformed worry can be even more destructive. I had no wish to present the Parents with this destruction. They were still reeling from the absence of the Husband and I made a decision - probably mistaken - to try to protect them for as long as possible. I am a parent myself and know just how much I hate it when my children hide things from me – this includes detentions, dirty mugs, matching socks, notes from school as well as anxieties and emotional concerns. However, I continued down my chosen course.

The younger generation would also need to know what was going on and I continued my role of Protector of Others for as long as possible. The Older Daughter was away and having problems of her own. These included a variety of health worries, problems with accommodation, opening bank accounts, obtaining identity cards, discovering burglaries and all the vagaries of living alone in a foreign country. My news was not the sort of news that one wishes to give over the phone to someone close who is living alone and abroad. However, prayers were answered when she announced that she was coming home for half term and my birthday. I had planned a pleasant day out for her: a neck and shoulder massage followed by lunch out in a local vegetarian restaurant by the river. I know it was supposed to be **my** birthday but that meant I could choose whatever I wanted to do and what I wanted to do was to treat the Older Daughter. But plans are there to be foiled and my plans were no exception.

First, there was the computer. I had ordered a new computer some time previously and was awaiting its delivery following a tortuous route from maker to deliverer that somehow involved Ireland and east London. At last, I had been offered a delivery date and time which had been narrowed down to "some time between 8 am and 6 pm on the aforementioned date."

There was nothing to be done so I rearranged lunch and resigned myself to waiting in all day. Thus it came as no surprise to me to be informed that the date of my assignation with Large-Needle was to be on that very same day. More stand-by plans were made to cover computer delivery and all was set.

Once the Older Daughter was home, I was able to tell her exactly why the plans had been changed and all that had precipitated my trip to ARDAC. She later admitted that she was very grateful to be able to see me in person and be reassured that things were not too bad. She had the massage to look forward to and then lunch somewhere, sometime. In the event, the computer arrived at 9 am, she departed for her massage and I set out once again for Hospital.

Thus it was that I celebrated the first part of my 52nd birthday back at ARDAC. When asked for my date of birth by the cheery nurse, I replied morosely, "Today!" Sympathy and congratulations mingled together and I entered the darkened room full of shiny machines and dutifully lay down on the bed. This was not the domain of the Frown, but that of a pleasant-faced and sympathetic woman who refused to allow a mere frown to cross her features. She administered the local anaesthetic and then produced Large-Needle. He was a most impressive character, powerfully built and with a penetrative stare that boded no good for the soft tissues of C-cup. Young Leader listened carefully to the explanations made by the Pleasant Smile. It was now or never and he finally made a decision. He gathered his troops around him once more and stood proudly to receive his fate.

Large-Needle poised himself above C-cup and

plunged into the depths. Full of his own importance, he plunged ever deeper – down and down, past the anaesthetised portions of C-cup and into fresh tissue that had never even been on nodding terms with any anaesthetic. My tiny and more or less controlled scream of pain frightened the Pleasant Smile and it disappeared briefly to be replaced by a look of deep concern. An apology was immediately forthcoming and Large-Needle was withdrawn. The pathetic results of his foray were held up for examination. It was a poor specimen and when placed in the appropriate container, it sank very gently to the bottom of the tube.

"I'm so sorry but I really think we need to go in again," apologised the Pleasant Smile as it reached across to the eyes that watched me with concern.

I held my breath and closed my eyes while Large-Needle made a second and less painful incursion. This time, the spoils were more acceptable to the Pleasant Smile and my ordeal was over. Pressing a large dressing tightly against C-cup, I gathered my clothes and emerged into the February day to continue with my birthday celebrations. One more week of waiting before the results would be clear.

<u>Chapter Six</u>

My results were due a week later and accordingly, I made my familiar journey to the stepped car park and glassy frontage of the Hospital. As I stepped inside, my nostrils were assailed with the smell that seems to be peculiar to that hospital. For the last few years, the Smell, although rather unpleasant, had been reassuring, comforting even, as I knew that I was being well cared for and that nothing would escape detection here. Today, for the first time, the Smell seemed threatening and overpowering. My resolve to be positive weakened and I began to regret that I had chosen to come alone. I had received many offers of company but had avoided them all. I did not wish to hurt anyone, but this was one appointment I wished to keep between me and the Great Italian. I knew I would be able to cope with the news, whatever it should be. One friend, a nurse, had asked me if I really believed it to be cancer and I remember replying with absolute confidence, "Yes."

This was not what she wanted to hear and set about trying to convince me otherwise. But I know my body and the Young Leader had been sending me pamphlets, posters and reminders for some time now. I listened and understood. I am blessed with a very strong Christian faith and knew that I would be given the wherewithal to cope. I had felt an enormous peace throughout the proceedings and indeed one friend had told me that I seemed to be almost radiant! This sounded rather too much as though the angels were lurking just the other side of the A3 and I made haste to rearrange my features into a more appropriate aspect. I dimmed down the external radiance and turned up the prayer support instead. This extended into a wide variety of locations, including four other countries, five different churches and even a synagogue or two.

The Smell penetrated my consciousness and I made my way to the cubicle once more.

The Great Italian entered accompanied by a woman wearing a badge. I peered rudely at her bosom and read the words 'Clinical Nurse Specialist". My heart sank. This was no chaperoning Staff Nurse. This Badge signified the need for support though whether for me or for the Great Italian, I did not know. The Badge smiled at me in a sympathetic manner and so it came as no surprise at all when the Great Italian took my hand and informed me gently that Young Leader had been discovered by Large Needle. I did indeed have cancer again. The Badge patted my knee and I took a deep breath to start the fight. Deep inside C-cup, Young Leader was celebrating his forthcoming exit into the world. His more fervent supporters cheered him on but those on the fringes began to feel a frisson of fear. Who would go? Who would be left behind? Older cells shivered and all were alert as they listened to the Great Italian. There could be no more radiotherapy as I had had my maximum dose. The cells cheered – no more burns! His next words filled them all with horror, "You will have to have a mastectomy!"

The Young Leader backed away from the hostility that was now advancing on him. No-one else had wanted to escape and now their hand had been forced. They were being forcibly ejected against their will and they knew exactly who to blame. Back in the tiny cubicle, I waited for the next move.

The Great Italian wanted me to have more tests so that he could make more exact plans. He left me with the Badge who patted my knee again and went to fetch the leaflet. When she returned after some time, I was seated on the bed, fully dressed again and considering my future. The Badge patted my knee, smiled gently and asked if I was feeling alright. I still felt calm and reassured her that all was fine. Then she launched the big one – who was at home for me? At this my stoicism leapt and ran from the room to be replaced by panic-induced tears as I informed her that there was only the Younger Daughter and that she needed me! More knee patting and a comforting arm as we considered the leaflet and my options. I was sent on my way to the blood tests with red and watery eyes and clutching various forms and, of course, the leaflet. Outside the cubicle, the row of waiting women flinched from my desperate face. It was their turn next.

I rounded the corner and approached the Blood Test Room. It was completely empty apart from a water cooler, several chairs and a pile of tattered magazines. A tall bespectacled man with a short-sleeved white coat buttoned high across the neck entered the room in front of me. The Spectacles gestured to the ticket machine and told me to take both a ticket and a seat. I was used to this. Apart from the seats and the magazines, it was just like the deli counter at the supermarket or the shoe department in the local John Lewis. I duly took a ticket and a seat. My ticket was numbered 16 and the red lit display above the door read 15. There was no-one else in the room. I had every confidence that the wait would be a short one.

The Spectacles came to the inner door and looked at me. He asked me what my number was and then compared my answer with the display above his head. It still read 15 so he went back inside the room and pressed a button. Magically, the number leapt to 16 and I half rose from my seat. The Spectacles returned and asked me for my number once again. I told him, showed him my ticket and then lowered myself back into the chair as he peered round the empty room as if looking for other possible contenders for the next in line.

"I think you may be next then," he finally admitted. I, too, looked around the empty waiting room and agreed that it was, in all probability, my turn next and I made my way into the inner sanctum. It had not been a good day for him and he proceeded to tell me all about it in no uncertain terms as he pierced my flesh with yet another needle. In the background, a Carole King song was playing. "It's too late" had accompanied my rejection by a former boyfriend, the departure for Australia of my best friend and several other significant moments in my life. I informed the Spectacles that this song always seemed to be playing at the really bad times of my life. "Is today bad then?" he asked without interest. I gestured to the forms that required me to make appointments for CT scans, bone scans, blood tests and the leaflet on mastectomy.

"Pretty bad," I replied and he sniffed, clearly refusing to believe that my day could possibly be worse than his. After confirming my name and date of birth several times, I left to make the aforesaid appointments in another part of the Hospital. This was easier said than done but I returned to the car park, assured that I would receive a letter very soon. I stopped en route home to take a call from the absent Husband who was deeply upset at my news. I managed to get home without further ado and made a few calls to anxiously waiting friends. Now was the time to tell the Parents and the Younger Daughter. Once more, I made my plans.

Chapter Seven

Two days later, I was driving down the suburban **A** road that led to my parents. I was anxious for them and my mind wandered as I tried to rehearse the words that would fill them with sorrow, horror and worry. I arrived to a flurry of hugs, kisses and lunch and then sat down with my cup of tea, steeling myself to utter those words. However, my parents had had a hard week and wanted to tell me all about it. I waited patiently for an auspicious opening but as they continued in their descriptions of the past week, I waited in vain. It transpired that they had been to a particularly difficult funeral and this did not seem to lead well into my own news. Funerals and breast cancer do not make good bedfellows when making announcements of this sort. So I waited a little longer.

My parents live in a retirement complex and it seemed that many of their neighbours had also had very hard weeks and I was treated to an account of each and every illness. This could have been my opening then but I did not wish to seem competitive and somehow, the time never seemed right. Time has a habit of taking over and mine was running out as I had to be home again to receive the laden bag, empty lunchbox and dirty P.E. kit of the Younger Daughter. Finally my mother noticed the time and said to me," It is so good to have such good news at the end of such an awful week." I was puzzled by this as I had not spoken more than a few words and wondered what this good news could be. I enquired.

"It's just so good to see you and know that you are in good health and here to cheer us up." I was touched by this but knew that this was it. This was my last chance and it could not have been a less auspicious opening but I ploughed ahead and plunged them headfirst into the horrors of their imaginations. I left them to a long and worried afternoon and a sleepless night, feeling awful for them but unable to help them as I caused this anxiety. I had unintentionally added to their pain by revealing my previous deceptions. Deceptions caused by not saying anything at an earlier stage and which now felt more like betrayal than protection.

Two down and three to go! The next morning, I telephoned to France to inform the Older Daughter. I chose my timing carefully as I knew that she would be spending the day with friends and I did not want her to receive this news whilst alone in her rooms. This was a little easier as she had already had some preparation but I felt for her as I left her to her own devices and turned my attention to the Younger Daughter, as yet ignorant of the blow that was about to fall on her. She came into my bed for the morning cuddle, half asleep and dreamy. I gentled her through the news in as light-hearted and positive way as possible and waited. She had recently supported her friend through similar circumstances and at once her Imagination leapt into the forefront of her mind and took over. I could see it running panic-stricken through her eyes as it sought a way to express itself. It rode on her shoulders, pushing them down and finally took her off to watch television but it would not keep quiet and it is doubtful whether she really saw the wild antics of Saturday morning Television presenters.

It took a further twenty four hours for her Imagination to finally pin her down and subdue her. Would she have to live alone, caring for herself? Worse, would she have to go and live elsewhere with the Absent Father and She-who-must-not-be-mentioned? Would the Older Sister have to give up University and look after her? Thankfully, her Imagination found its way to her tongue and she confessed her fears. I lost no time in assuring her that I had no intention of making a permanent disappearance from her life and sought assurances from the Absent Husband that he would look after her in her own home should it be otherwise. Last but in no way least, I telephoned the In-Laws and managed to ruin their Sunday too. I recalled seeing the grey faces of my mother and mother-in-law as they bent over my bed nineteen years previously, shocked to the very helpless core by the diagnosis of cancer. I had not wanted to repeat that experience ever again and yet here I was, forcing the people I loved most to reach down into those depths and face those horrors with me. Life moved on and we all remained with our own thoughts deep inside, sharing them whenever necessary.

Meanwhile, the letter had arrived from the Hospital with my appointment dates and times for the scans. I was due to have two scans – a CT scan and a bone scan and timing was of the essence. The bone scan required an injection followed by a three hour wait punctuated with frequent drinks followed by the scan. The CT scan required an injection followed by an hour's wait and then the scan. I had hoped for a sandwich appointment with the CT scan fitted neatly into the three hour wait. However, sandwiches were off the menu and the more modern stacking had taken its place with the bone scan to follow the CT scan and this meant I was in line for a very long day. The indefatigable J came to the rescue and promised her services as chauffeur, companion and comforter and I accepted with unaccustomed alacrity.

We duly arrived at the Hospital armed with books, magazines and sandwiches and made our way to the X-ray department. The waiting room was already full, a fact that never ceases to fill me with sadness and horror that so many people are undergoing these traumas. We took the only two available seats which were in a corner either side of the water dispenser. If you wish to make friends in the scanning department, then this is the place to sit. All around me, track-suited people sat clutching their polystyrene cups. Each of us had our instructions and that was to drink the required number of cups of water prior to the scan. My whispered conversations with J were continuously interrupted by a stream of apologetic cup-clutchers as we drank our way to the bottom of the dispenser. I had accepted the proffered cup with considerable trepidation as she informed me that my requirement was six cups. I recalled only too well the bladder-clenching days of a previous bone scan and several ante-natal scans where the scanners were rolled with ever increasing pressure over my groaning body and the prospect of sudden incontinence loomed large though never, thankfully, achieved. Nervously, I asked if I were permitted to go to the loo during my wait and was greatly relieved to be told that it was perfectly alright to do so.

Now I like drinking water and do so a great deal but not normally in such a short space of time and I was beginning to feel bloated and uncomfortable as I drank my way through my allotted portion. The waiting room emptied slowly but then, six cups of water and three loo visits later I was summoned for the injection. A cannula was placed in my arm following comments about the size of my veins (A Good Thing), the misfortune of my situation (A Bad Thing) and the need to remember to keep the cannula in after the scan ready for my next injection (A Necessary Thing). I was then asked to wait just outside the room for a short while. Obediently I found a chair, waved to J through the adjoining windows and sat and waited. After half an hour I gave up sitting alone and walked back round the corner to J so that we could both have some company. They would be able to find me when my time finally came.

At last my name was called by a harassed looking nurse who gestured to me to remain seated and that I would have another wait as an Emergency had arrived. The Emergency's husband sat, bowed and hunched in my recently vacated seat and I spared him a prayer as I sat back in my chair. I glanced at the watch I had put in my handbag, following the injunction to wear no metal and realised that it was perilously close to the time for my bone scan injection. Suddenly, my name was called with some urgency and I leapt to my feet. I was told to run round to Nuclear Medicine and have the injection for the bone scan and to make it fast! I obeyed but refrained from running, whether from some long buried reaction to the school rule of no running in the corridor, or the more likely feeling that running was neither comfortable nor seemly. I walked but walked fast and was whisked in through the electronic doors that hid the Nuclear Medicine Department.

A kindly New Zealander took my particulars and proceeded to ask me a few questions, the most memorable of which was, "Could you possibly be pregnant?" I laughed and pointed out my age – 52. He assured me that it was more than possible to be pregnant at 52 and he repeated the question. I sought more proof. "I don't have a live-in Husband," I offered. But that was apparently no proof either as many women who did not have certificated Husbands still managed to become pregnant. I could see him wondering if they ought to offer sex education lessons prior to bone scans as I searched for yet further proof of my definitely non-pregnant status.

Triumphantly, I played my trump card," I haven't had a period for five years." I cried. "I am well and truly post-menopausal." He still did not look convinced but a glance at his watch informed him that he had to accept my word. As he plugged the needle into my cannula, he informed me that I would now be radioactive and should avoid pregnant women and small children. I was to wait for three hours during which time I could have my lunch and drink at least two litres of water. He forestalled my next and obvious question by instructing me to visit the loo as often as possible so that I could flush the radioactive fluid through my whole body. I was then reminded to hurry back for my CT scan before I lost yet another slot. I didn't meet any pregnant women or small children on the short but speedy walk back to my waiting room. The nurses were waiting for me and I was hustled in for yet another injection.

This would apparently give me a very hot flush and a feeling that I desperately needed the loo which I was assured would not actually be the case. The six cups of water assured me otherwise and I made a quick and apologetic dash up and down the now familiar corridor before taking my place on the couch. The machine arched above me, flashing important sounding but coded messages to the waiting staff as the injection coursed through me.

Their predictions were indeed right, but the hot and burning sensations soon passed along with the aforesaid desire for the loo. This time, I remained still and all was well. Music filled the room and I lay watching the moving arch and the flashing codes, obediently holding and releasing my breath when so instructed by a combination of a disembodied voice and a series of cartoon faces in the LED display above me. My soft tissues shuddered as the machine passed over them, hoping against hope that the cell rebellion inspired by the Young Leader had not spread elsewhere.

Twenty minutes later, I staggered into the waiting room feeling disorientated and shivering with a terrible coldness. I still do not understand that reaction which was similar to the one I usually experience after anaesthetic. J took one look at me and hustled me out of the waiting room and down to the restaurant for warmth and nourishment. The shivering slowly wore off and we ate our sandwiches accompanied by the monotonous kicking of the vending machine. This seemed to be the only way it could be persuaded to give up its treasures but it was irritating and intrusive and so we elected to take a stroll round the grounds in the February sunshine. We hadn't bargained for the biting February wind and our stroll was short. It took in only the road to the car park before we turned our footsteps to the entrance again and sought refuge in the little coffee shop. We sat in companionable silence with our books and coffees, broken only by my frequent visits to both water dispenser and toilet as I forced my way through a further two litres of water.

The three hours seemed interminable but eventually, we made our way back up to Nuclear Medicine for the final act of the day. The wait was reasonably short this time and I soon found myself in an enormous and antiseptic looking room dominated by the scanning machine. I lay on the bed and immediately my feet were tied together. My wrists were placed in a huge rubber band and my head turned to one side. I began to wonder if I had wandered into some weird and sadistic dream but reality soon hit me as the bed was slowly raised until I was nose to nose with the Scanner. I felt claustrophobic and somewhat panicky as I surveyed the machine out of the corner of my eye. Surely the vast mound of my stomach would not fit through that small space. My back, already prone to arthritic grumblings, began to complain vociferously and I seriously doubted that I could remain in that position for five minutes let alone for the threatened forty five minutes. The operator pressed a button, the Scanner rumbled into life and I fought down an urgent need to scream. I tried relaxing – no good. I tried counting – no good.

The operator left the room after telling me that I could now look straight upwards. This was easier on the still complaining back but put me on rather more intimate terms with the arched machine. I closed my eyes and prayed as the machine rumbled its way down my body. I prayed for myself, for my family and friends and for all those who had to lie on this very couch at other times on other days. The operator returned and the Scanner stuttered to a halt. The forty five minutes had only been in actual fact, twenty five minutes and my wrists and feet were released from their bondage as the operator asked me a few pertinent questions. I steeled myself for the one about being pregnant but it did not arise, replaced by the more frightening, "Have you had pains in your bones or joints recently?" I reviewed my body joint by joint and confessed to problems with spine, thumbs, toes, hips, elbows, shoulders and not forgetting the neck. I muttered the word 'osteoarthritis' at him but watched him ticking his chart with the red biro with mounting horror. He then asked me about previous breast surgery and/or radiotherapy and I crawled off the couch convinced that the scan had revealed far more than I had expected. The soothing J assured me that they were just routine questions and she whisked me back to the car and home. It was time to do what I was learning to do best – wait!

Chapter Eight

I had made two appointments at clinic to receive my results. One was for two weeks hence and was also the night before I was due to take twenty brownies away for the weekend – not the best timing in the world. I had, however, made a provisional appointment for the week before just in case the results were through earlier. I was to finish my morning's work at midday and then telephone the hospital to see if the results of all the tests were back in clinic. The faithful J was ready and waiting to accompany me on this journey into the unknown.

The day duly arrived and I made every effort not to be too distracted as I listened to readers, oversaw the sewing of felt butterflies and rabbits, did my playground duty and guided a small group through the vagaries of open number lines. At midday, I closeted myself in the staffroom and rang the Hospital. The results were in. Accompanied to the gate by my wonderful job share, I confessed to a deep anxiety beneath my easygoing exterior. She hugged me warmly and sent me on my way to wait for J and yet another trip to the very familiar glass entrance.

A nervous wait later, I was once again

ensconced in a tiny cubicle, inadequately wrapped in a gown and sitting on the bed, waiting. The Peace which had filled me for so long took one look at my face and ran headlong out of the door, leaving my mind wide open to the invasion of the much less friendly but alliterative cousin, Panic. I suddenly felt overwhelmed with fear. It was my usual bête noir, the fear of the unknown. I considered my options. If the tests proved negative, then I was facing radical surgery followed by, at the very least, a five year course of Tamoxifen. If the tests proved positive, then immediate surgery was out of the question and instead I would probably undergo chemotherapy, hormone treatment and then possibly surgery if necessary. I knew that I would be able to cope with either situation, but the not knowing was proving extremely hard to cope with.

Suddenly the door opened and the Great Italian entered, flanked by a staff nurse. For one awful moment I really thought I was going to throw up on the floor and add humiliation and a shoe cleaning bill to my burdens.

I recalled a previous appointment many years before following yet another scare and mysterious mammogram results when I waited for an hour in the huge waiting room, my nerves jangling and sure I must have missed my name. I was finally ushered into a cubicle where I waited shivering with cold and fear for forty minutes alone with my thoughts. At last a young doctor entered clutching my notes and results. He laid them face up on the chair and began to prod. Suddenly, he flipped the papers over so that the results were no longer visible and asked me where the lump had been last time. Last time? Was this then the next time? By now, I was seriously worried and in a state of highly charged tension. After much frowning, prodding and consultation of my notes which he held firmly away from me, he announced that all was well and that I could go away for another year.

"Do you mean that you knew my results were clear all the time?" I shouted.

The doctor looked somewhat taken aback by the ferocity of my tones but confirmed my suppositions. I leapt off the bed, gown flying, eyes flashing and all nerves gone. "Sit down there!" I commanded him. He had a nurse to protect him but she merely waited to one side while I towered above the now cowering doctor.

"Don't you ever do that again," I yelled as though he were a recalcitrant five year old. In no uncertain terms, I gave him a lesson in patient care, pointing out the need to reassure the anxious patient as soon as possible after entering the room and to be aware of the possible implications of suddenly appearing to hide results. He had the good grace to apologise before fleeing to the sanctuary afforded by the inner sanctum. The nurse clapped me quietly before she too disappeared to make my next annual appointment.

But my present situation was different. The Great Italian was a kind and understanding man who knew only too well what it was like to be on the receiving end of the doctor-patient relationship.

Not for him the delaying tactics of his juniors. As he approached and shook my hand, he was already telling me that my scans and blood tests had not revealed any further spread of cancer. If he was surprised by the firmness of my grip or the warmth of my thank you, he did not show it but continued on with the announcement that I would almost certainly now be having a mastectomy.

Almost? The word jumped at me and I listened carefully as he informed me that the bone scan had revealed some 'lively activity on a rib' and that he wished me to have an immediate X-ray before finally committing himself to surgery. I asked for his opinion on the possibility of doing a bilateral mastectomy, thus removing both breasts at once. He sank into a chair fanning himself as if in shock. His humour put me at ease as he informed me that medically it was not considered necessary and that it would only be on aesthetic grounds that he could consider this option. However, he was not prepared to put me through such an operation unnecessarily but promised me that if I could not cope with lopsided life, that he would remove the other breast in years to come.

I thanked him yet again and, clutching the appropriate form, made my way up to X-ray.

The wait here was mercifully short but the light hearted banter between myself and J was smothered by the appearance of a very sick little boy in a wheelchair. The full realisation of my position hit me and I felt very grateful for small mercies. Some minutes later, holding my X-ray and trying to work out the implications of the shadowy area on the rib, I returned to clinic. I informed J that she had now seen parts of me unseen before by any friend, parts that were usually hidden by layers of flesh and material – my very bones. Somehow that didn't fill her with the awe and gratitude I felt it deserved, but nothing could shake my buoyant mood as I waited outside clinic for the opinion of the Great Italian. He confirmed that it did not look serious and so once again I left the Hospital, armed with an appointment for a pre – admission check-up and a probable date for surgery three weeks hence.

I was no sooner in the car than my texting fingers hit the buttons of my mobile phone as I blasted my good news around family and friends. Over the next few days, as the news percolated to the outer fringes of my groups, I was hugged, congratulated, celebrated and cheered. Without fail, people were overjoyed and simultaneously horrified at their joy. After all, I still had cancer and was facing major and disfiguring surgery followed by as yet unknown treatments. But it hadn't spread and that in itself was cause for joy and prayerful thanks.

Time to make more plans.

Chapter Nine

My plans centred round my Brother from the North as he had volunteered to come down and look after the Younger Daughter during my stay in Hospital. We have an unusual relationship it would seem, my Brother from the North and I: we like each other! Many's the time I have been plunged into incomprehension as my friends have related tales of sibling dislike and competitiveness; of fights over parental funerals; of legal and moral battles over money and property; of an inability to co-exist except under extreme duress. I have always liked and loved my Brother from the North. Even as children, although we would fight physically, we would remain staunch allies in the face of opposition.

I remember during the sixties, when life was dominated by fear of nuclear attack and the Four-Minute Warning, that my only wish was that when that dreaded Warning came, I could be with my brother to protect him and keep him from being fearful. We no longer fight at all but continue to support each other through thick and thin and there had been quite a lot of both thick and thin in both our lives in recent years. A sort of Warning had sounded now in my life and it was his turn to come to the rescue and protect me. He cancelled his clinics, rearranged his life and prepared to come to London for a week.

Meanwhile, I set about reorganising my life. I delegated some of my duties as before; cut short the Brownie term; compiled a list of important phone numbers for my Brother's information and wrote a detailed list of daily requirements for the Younger Daughter and the two cats. I notified the school that I would be absent for a while and all was ready. The operation had been scheduled for the last week of the Spring term and the many after-school activities undertaken by the Younger Daughter would have finished before that date so that chauffeuring duties would be kept to a minimum. I was booked in for a five-night stay and was due out of hospital on the first day of the Easter holidays – all very convenient.

However, before then, I had yet another visit to the Hospital for my pre-admissions checks. The next Wednesday morning found me back up in the misnamed Rapid Diagnostic Unit. An hour after my arrival I had finished reading my paper, attempted the Times crossword (succeeding only in completing three clues), studied my fellow patients with some curiosity and tried (and failed) to understand why everyone else seemed to be called and yet I was still waiting.

At last, my name was called and I was ushered into a large examination room dominated by a bed and a computer. The computer was attended by a young tired looking man whom I assumed to be a doctor but who looked more like an escapee from the City, with his blue striped shirt and red braces. The Red Braces untangled themselves from a stethoscope and half rose from the swivel seat as I entered. Gesturing to me to take the other chair, they lowered themselves tiredly into their seat again and my examination began. The first question was easy: What was the date of my proposed admission. I informed the Red Braces that the admission date was the 28th March with surgery on 29th March. The Red Braces looked confused and swivelled the computer round for easier contemplation. There ensued a few minutes of intense study combined with deep sighing and then the Red Braces sat back in their chair, "You shouldn't be in this room at all. Wrong dates." I protested that I had already waited an hour to be seen and pleaded with the Red Braces to find some way of changing things so that I could be in the right room after all.

After much study of the screen, I was informed that as my surgery date was for the 28th March, I should really be seeing another doctor but that this one would try his best to accommodate me. I gently pointed out that my surgery date was the 29th March and that it was my admission date that was the 28th. Apparently, that meant that I was, after all, in the right room and the examination continued.

All went well for a while until we reached the thorny issue of the 'lively activity' on the rib. I was informed that I would have to go and have a chest x-ray before completing my check–in procedure. I could see no reason for an unnecessary x-ray and made my feelings as clear as possible. The Red Braces insisted that such an x-ray was absolutely essential but I continued to plead my case, assuring them that I had already had a chest x-ray to check out the 'lively activity'. Apparently, this information had not yet been transferred to my electronic notes but I won my case and we settled down to further questioning.

Once this was completed to the satisfaction of the Red Braces, we turned to another area of the form, as I needed to sign what was called 'informed consent'. This consisted of Red Braces informing me of all the potentially fatal or near fatal problems that could arise during or after surgery. The list seemed endless and rather frightening but I agreed to sign the form and so the correct pages were duly printed and laid in front of me. Red Braces took up his pen and signed his part of the form with a flourish. He then considered his handiwork and realised that he had signed the part of the form marked 'patient consent'. Apologies were made and excuses given, blaming a new set-up on electronic forms as opposed to other types of paperwork. The name was duly scribbled out and I signed and dated both forms in the correct space. Red Braces confirmed my signature and I was transferred to the bed for a physical examination. Red Braces had an unusual technique, which involved the use of knuckles, rather than fingers, thus making me feel more like a piece of bread dough than a human being.

However, a few questions later, I was released back into the system and sent downstairs for more blood tests. My kindly nurse advised me to have coffee after the tests, as there would be some delay before the next round of check-ups. Clutching several blood test forms and my somewhat creased newspaper, I went downstairs once more.

This time, the room was fairly full and I continued my struggle with the crossword whilst keeping a vigilant eye on the red display above the door. At last, my number was called and I made my way into the little room to find the Spectacles in a very bad temper. It appeared that several errors had been reported concerning inadequate labelling of tubes. I made sure that all my tubes were well labelled before leaving for my well-earned coffee. I had half an hour to kill, so I sat back with the aforementioned coffee, the recalcitrant crossword and a willing pen. I was halfway through the coffee and no further on with the crossword when I dropped the newspaper. To my horror, I found that a single blood test form had taken refuge among its pages and had therefore been overlooked.

I glanced at my watch, swallowed the remains of my polystyrene coffee and hastened back to the Blood test room, which was still quite full. I cowered in the corner, hoping against hope that I would manage to avoid the Spectacles. My luck was in and I slipped into another corner and explained my predicament. My elbow crease was already bandaged following the first test and so this second needle was inserted in the back of my hand. My feelings of relief at avoiding the Spectacles were short-lived as yet another complaint was made concerning a poorly labelled tube. Who was the culprit this time? None other than the very person engaged in piercing my veins. She had not even asked for my date of birth yet and I was quick to give her that information several times, watching while she wrote it correctly on my tube. Shielding my face with my newspaper as though I was trying to avoid media attention rather than the gaze of the Spectacles, I left the Blood Test room for the last time and returned to ARDAC.

The kindly nurse collected me from the waiting room and showed me into a vast room full of electronic equipment, scanners and screens. Once more deprived of my upper garments, I submitted to an ECG. The electrodes were then removed and I was asked to wait for a blood pressure check. The kindly nurse left the room and I was left alone among the stainless steel and flashing lights. For ten minutes, I sat on the edge of the bed and shivered, as I had no gown to cover my modesty or my goose bumps. By the time the kindly nurse returned, I was cold and I had had enough of ARDAC.

Unsurprisingly, my blood pressure was much raised and I was dismissed with the instructions to get two more readings taken at my GP surgery and to phone them through before my admission. The kindly nurse delivered dire warnings of the consequences of high blood pressure at surgery, not the least of which was the information that the operation might well not take place if my BP was too high. I left the Hospital, cold, tired and confused and returned home to attempt to make two appointments with Dr and/or nurse for blood pressure checks the following week. This was easier said than done but at last I was successful and set about trying to keep calm for the next few days.

Calmness was not uppermost in my mind by the time I reached the consulting room as the waiting room had been disturbed by doctors switching on the radio, filling the space with noise and then electric light. They stamped into their rooms and flung bags on their desks and so it was with some surprise that I noted a reduction in my blood pressure reading. This was probably due to the reading being taken with a wide cuff and I decided that in future, I would insist on a wide cuff. A change of tablets and one further reading later that week and I was finally ready to enter the Hospital as an in-patient once again.

Chapter Ten

My first hurdle was to succeed in the bed lottery. I was to ring the Hospital at 9 am on the Sunday morning to see if a bed was still available. This I duly did with my heart in my mouth. All those careful plans could still go astray but the operation was obviously meant to be and a bed was available as predicted. At church that morning, several people asked me if I was better, having read my name on the prayer list. I informed them that I was due to go in to Hospital that very afternoon. I felt very much cared for and loved and supported. The Younger Daughter decided to accompany us in the afternoon and we set off with a packed bag full of wash things, books, puzzle books, cd player and, regrettably, only one night T-shirt. Why regrettably? Time will tell.

As we entered the great glass portals once again, I sensed a difference to the Hospital. The massive entrance area was usually teeming with people: patients waiting for transport home; ambulance and taxi drivers looking for people to take home; white coated, stethoscope-wielding doctors in a hurry; blue-uniformed nurses clutching sheaves of forms; bewildered visitors wandering in a daze as they sought the right department; green-sashed volunteers giving gentle directions and kindly help. But today, the whole area was completely empty. The grills to the little shop and the pharmacy were closed, the reception desks unattended and neither patient nor professional walked the usually busy floor. Something else was also missing – that awful Smell had glanced at the calendar and realised that it was Sunday. It had taken the day off and vanished into the March sunshine to kick its heels far away from those who wrinkled up their noses in its presence. It had left behind a vague imprint on the air as if to remind all comers that it was not so very far away and would be back. I welcomed its absence as we continued our journey through the Hospital.

Confidently, we made our way towards the stairs and the arrowed signs to the wards. A yellow sign pointed up and so up we went. No sign of the required ward and no more signs but, knowing it was on the second floor, up we went again. Still no sign of the right ward and puzzlement began to crease our hitherto unmarked faces. The Brother from the North ran up another flight of stairs but returned shaking his head. We ventured round an unpromising corner and found ourselves in a long bare corridor, littered with abandoned trolleys, piles of dustsheets and tins of an unprepossessing coloured paint. We returned to the stairs and descended once again to the empty and echoing entrance hall. It was then that I noticed another yellow sign, this time pointing along the lower corridor to another wing. We followed the pointing arrow and then climbed another two flights of stairs. Still no ward. There were one or two other wards in the vicinity but not mine. There were no nurses, doctors, orderlies, cleaners or any other signs of life. The Brother from the North disappeared into a ward that did exist and finally returned with instructions.

At last, we reached the right destination and were welcomed warmly before being shown into a four-bedded ward with three occupants and an empty, crisp-sheeted bed by the window.

I was given a cup of tea and told to make myself comfortable for a minute or so and the Welcome vanished into the corridor. We sat on the bed and gazed out of the window, aware that we were being perused by the other occupants, shielded by their headphones, bouquets and bedside cabinets awash with jugs and books and papers. We sat and we waited. And waited. Finally, the Welcome returned armed with a clipboard full of questions. She invited me to accompany her into a quiet room to complete the questionnaires and the Brother from the North came with us, leaving the Younger Daughter alone on my bed. I promised that we wouldn't be too long and left her with many a backward glance of anxiety. The patient in the opposite bed gave me a reassuring nod and I followed in the wake of the Welcome. Many questions later, we returned to the ward to find the Younger Daughter watching what appeared to be my own personal television. The opposite bed had explained its use to her and was still smiling encouragingly.

I felt more relaxed now and settled in to the routine of admission. The plastic name bracelets were brought to me and my name, date of birth and number were checked. The first bracelet was fixed irremovably round my left wrist and then the first of many little humiliations occurred as the second bracelet refused to accept its intended lowly position round my ankle. It fought long and hard for its rightful place and was finally accorded the position of right wrist bracelet. It was then the turn of the two red bracelets. It was with considerable anxiety that I viewed the written label which read '**penicillen**'. I had to hope that this was a spelling error and not an allergy to an unknown drug. The second red bracelet conceded defeat without a struggle and took its place on my right wrist without so much as a glance at my deeply embarrassed and obviously over large ankle.

The Welcome disappeared in search of further humiliations and a phone number for the ward, promising a speedy return. This proved to be an empty promise as it was some time before she returned with a packet of extra large support stockings and no phone number. Dinner was smelt in the corridors and the Brother from the North and the Younger Daughter decided to leave me to it. I accompanied them down to the ground floor so that I could buy my patient phone card. I decided against leaving a trail of crumbs so that I could find my way back again and concentrated on memorising the route instead. It turned out to be surprisingly easy and so I waved goodbye to my anxious looking daughter and sibling and went back up to the ward to eat my dinner, suss out my fellow patients and wait for the anaesthetist's rounds.

He turned out to be young and gorgeous and very sympathetic. I explained my usual reactions to anaesthetic to him. Firstly, I was always sick following surgery and he made haste to reassure me that I would be given an appropriate cocktail of drugs to ease this problem. Secondly, I always came round in the recovery room to find myself shuddering with cold. My last operation, a minor one on my eye, had been in a private hospital in Surrey and I had wakened from surgery shaking almost uncontrollably and apparently unable to signal this fact to the nurses in attendance. Looking back now, I can see that maybe the shuddering just felt violent and was not evident to the hovering nurses. At the time, I feared that I would shake myself off the bed. I finally managed to draw attention to my plight and in a few moments, I was shrouded in heated duvets and blankets. Gradually, the shivering stopped and I began my speedy road to recovery. The gorgeous young anaesthetist assured me that this would all be taken into account. Then he painted my left shoulder with yellow paint and drew a circle above my left breast. There followed a slightly surreal conversation as he explained that the painting was to guarantee that the surgeon would remove the right breast and I contended that it should be the left breast. Linguistic misunderstandings were rectified and I relaxed again.

My next visitor was one of the wonderful Js who came bearing gifts and encouragements and to ensure that I had everything I needed. She wished me well and departed, leaving me to fathom out the television and to settle into institution life. The television was an amazing example of modern technology. A flat screen hung poised above the bed, ready to be pulled down whenever required. Touch screen buttons gave a choice of channels and settings and headphones dangled spider-like from the handle so that no-one else would have to listen to the same programmes. Privacy and entertainment in one electronic package. Beside the bed, lay my own personal phone with its own personal number. No more waiting for the telephone trolley to be trundled round the ward or into the day room. No more desperate searching for coins as you tried to inform family and friends of your latest update and were cut off mid-sentence, leaving them at best, puzzled, and at worst, frightened by unfinished phrases. No more lying helpless in bed and listening to the endless ringing of the unanswered phone and wondering if it might just have been for you. All these modern additions combined to make the life of a hospital in-patient just a little more bearable.

I lay back on my starched sheets and considered my co-patients. The kind one opposite was wearing a wonderful hat in soft felt covered with rather South American looking patterns. This Hat had a mind of its own and its favourite position was seated rather rakishly astride one eyebrow. Its owner preferred the more traditional straight down above both ears. The Hat slid happily over the head that had been shaved against the effects of chemotherapy and resisted all efforts to keep it controlled. The Hat guided me in the routine of the ward and we chatted in a desultory fashion in between visits from nurses, orderlies and her family who used the occasion to watch television and send text messages while sprawled comfortably across her bed. I thought again how hospital life had changed over the years, recalling the sharp barks of Sister if she found anyone sitting on a bed; the misery of watching daytime television with the sound turned up for the benefit of the old lady in bed three who was sleeping the sleep of the heavily drugged anyway; the irritation of trying to watch a programme whilst nurses and doctors poked and prodded or uneasy relatives laughed too loudly.

Diagonally opposite, the patient was surrounded by flowers and interesting looking bottles and packets. She seemed to be surgically attached to her television via the umbilical headphones and only spoke to say goodbye when she left the next day. The patient next door to me had been on an outing for the day, prior to her discharge, and was rather tired so she, too, was quiet. I didn't mind the peace and quiet of the ward and I had the Hat and the television for company.

Time moved on and I felt rather like a condemned prisoner as I ate my last meal, drank my last hot drink and just managed to hang on to a small glass of water ready for my blood pressure tablet early next morning. Temperatures were taken, blood pressures recorded, medicines administered where necessary, teeth were cleaned and lights were turned off. We were left with the soft glow of the diagonally opposite television and our thoughts.

Deep in C-cup, the Young Leader made his apologetic peace with the rest of the cells as they prepared for their last night together. Tomorrow was fast approaching and all his plans would come to fruition. Older, wiser cells could see the flaws in these plans but wisely forbore to enlighten him, instead making their own preparations for the final separation. I said a fond goodnight to C-cup and then I slept.

Chapter Eleven

A pale grey light penetrated my sleeping brain and I struggled to remember where I was. The sight of a nurse bending over me to remind me to take my blood pressure tablet with just one swallow of water soon brought me into full consciousness and I duly took my tablet. The day was quiet and misty outside but with a promise that the sun would break through eventually. As the smells of hot toast filled the ward, I decided to avoid the sight of others eating their breakfast by going to get washed and robe myself in the delightful hospital gown. I returned quickly to fetch my dressing gown so that I could retain a little dignity when coming back into the ward. Hospital gowns gape widely across the back and my back was wider than most so I was in for a very wide display of my nether regions. My catwalk entrance in the day's most up-to-date fashion brought a smattering of applause from my audience who then watched with increasing fascination as I did battle with the surgical support hose. These were long white elasticised stockings designed to prevent blood clots both during and after surgery. I have rarely worn tights for the last few years as the attempts to put them on have usually reduced me to a sweating, puffing and often tearful wreck.

I took the enemy out of the bag marked **extra large** and viewed them with suspicion. They did not look extra large to me. I examined my legs. They, on the other hand, certainly did look extra large. I separated one stocking from its intimate relationship with the other and unfolded it slowly. The instructions on the packet informed me that I must find the hole at the toe, roll the stocking down to that hole and gently insert my foot. This was easier said (or written) than done as the elastic was very strong. The finding the hole bit was fairly straightforward although I was a little confused by the appearance of **two** holes. However, I correctly identified the toe hole and then fought to roll down the stocking. This was finally achieved and I sat on my chair gazing from the rolled up elastic nest in one hand, to the foot at the other end of my extra large leg. The audience straightened their pillows, sat up a little and abandoned all pretence of not watching my struggles. I leant over to insert the toe as instructed. My first problem was that I couldn't reach my toe.

The extra large leg was accompanied by an extra large stomach which was obviously feeling rather envious of the attention centred on its lower neighbour. It bundled itself up and created a barrier between me and my foot that seemed insurmountable. This was no new problem to me and was, indeed, the reason for not wearing tights. However, a struggle in the privacy of my own bedroom which usually involved me lying on the floor with one leg at right angles to the other, was one thing, but to fight such a battle from a deep armchair wedged between a high-sided bed and a brick wall, was quite another. Added to this, was the pressure created by my fascinated audience. I attempted to move the extra large stomach to one side and attacked my foot from a different angle. This had some success and I was finally able to insert my toe into the rolled down stocking. I sat up, purple in the face and breathing heavily, perused the instructions and considered my next move. This was to gently roll the stocking up the leg. It all sounded so easy but the elastic wasn't going to give in that easily and fought a valiant fight all the way to the knee.

I sat back, exhausted but triumphant, and my audience nodded appreciatively. The Hat smiled sympathetically and then reminded me that I still had one stocking left to go. Sighing deeply, I picked up the remaining stocking and prepared once more to do battle. I will leave the ensuing struggle to the imagination but came through with flying, if a little tattered, colours. My audience immediately pretended that they had not, after all, been watching me but had just been stretching their backs, watching the weather through the window beside me or looking at the cards on my bedside table. I was very glad that I would be spending the rest of the day having a lie-down.

Light relief came in the form of a nurse with a clipboard. I willingly confirmed my name, date of birth and hospital number; agreed that I was allergic to the correctly spelt Penicillin; acknowledged that I had not eaten since the previous evening and that I was correctly garbed for my outing to the theatre and then faltered at the next question. This was concerning jewellery. I taped my rings as instructed and then pondered the question, "I see you have no earrings in. Do you have any jewellery elsewhere?" I made a mental search of my body and then asked, "What exactly do you mean?"

Laughing, the nurse informed me that she was checking on body piercings. I made another mental and quite unnecessary sweep of my body and confirmed that I had no piercings anywhere else. Suddenly, earrings sounded rather barbaric. The jolly nurse disappeared with the paperwork and left me to my thoughts.

These were soon interrupted by another, though more serious, clipboard. Once again, I confirmed my name, date of birth and number. Once again, I discussed my recent dietary habits and fashion sense, displayed my taped finger and bare ears and informed her that I had no piercings anywhere else. She left, a little annoyed that I had pre-empted most of her questions, but still armed with clipboard, pen and information. Back to my thoughts once again. I was feeling very calm and positive about my forthcoming operation. If the long list of possible disasters signed up to in the deeper reaches of the hospital with Red Braces, wandered across my mind, I banished them very quickly. Young Leader was on his way out of my body and that was all that mattered. If he had to take unwilling companions with him, then so be it. I prayed a silent prayer for the surgeons and the gorgeous young anaesthetist and sat back to wait.

Right on cue, a small commotion appeared in the ward, consisting of the jolly nurse, a suited porter, a clipboard and a trolley. With some difficulty, I manoeuvred myself onto the trolley, waved farewell to my erstwhile audience and amidst the cries of 'good luck', the commotion and I left the ward.

Once on our way, I began to wonder if the suited porter was actually trained for the job as the trolley bounced off a wall, narrowly missed an orderly with her arms full of sheets, slewed tantalisingly towards a lift and finally crashed through the double doors marked **theatre**.

I found myself in a room full of humming machines and shelves full of mysterious bottles and packages. I glanced at the clock which informed me that it was seven o'clock. This surprised me as I had left the ward just before eight and we had travelled no more than a hundred yards. I did not recall time travel in the wild careering down the short corridors. Two green capped and green gowned figures appeared silently at my side. Their approach had been softened by the matching green covers on their shoes but my heart sank when I noticed that they were both clutching clipboards. The female green cap informed me that she was assisting the anaesthetist and just wanted to check on my propensity for nausea and shuddering as well as allergies. She viewed the red bracelet with a slight frown as she struggled to recall spellings and then her face cleared and she ticked something on the clipboard. She yawned hugely and glanced at the clock. Taken by surprise at the earliness of the hour, she consulted first her watch, which read the same and then the male green cap, who informed her that it was eight o'clock not seven. Our confusion was cleared when we realised that the clocks had gone forward during the night but that these clocks had been missed.

The male green cap approached me with his clipboard. Unasked, I informed him of my name, date of birth and number and that I was correctly attired, unfed and in possession of no body piercings. Laughing, he advised the female green cap that she probably had time for a coffee break as **his** clipboard ran to several pages. Together, we raced through the answers as his pen ticked and crossed in an arbitrary fashion. We agreed that paperwork was the bugbear of the NHS and, indeed, could bring about the downfall of civilisation.

Three pages later, he abandoned the clipboard and started rummaging in a drawer. I knew the countdown time was coming. This is the moment when a needle is inserted into your hand and you are asked to count backwards from ten. At number ten, I always felt as though the anaesthetic would not take effect before I reached one and that the whole operation would take place while I was still conscious. By number five, I usually began to panic a bit because I never felt as sleepy as I was expecting to feel. I never reached number four. In spite of the panic bit, I quite liked this part as it gave me a sense of adventure. Would this be the time I reached number four or maybe even the more daring number three? Green cap approached me again. "I'm just going to give you something to make you feel happy," he reassured me and promptly did so.

Chapter Twelve

As I struggled up through the layers of consciousness that seemed to pressing down on me, I became aware of two things. Firstly, I seemed to have been deprived of my countdown. I had been misled by the offer of happiness which had knocked me out without the need for my rocket launching practice.   Secondly, a disembodied voice was announcing to all listeners that my blood pressure was extremely low. This did not sound at all likely as I suffer from high blood pressure and, indeed, had nearly missed the operation due to the height of the said blood pressure. I wondered if I was actually me after all or had I been swapped with some other patient?   Then I heard my name being called, gently at first and then more and more insistently until I reluctantly opened my eyes. The bright lights directly above my head bored into my eyes and I closed them again with much relief. The voice started up again and peering through semi-closed eyelids, I could just make out that it was attached to a head and green-clad body.   I acknowledged that I was awake and breathing and was told to go back to sleep for a while. I needed no second telling and obediently drifted off into a sleep peopled with green headless beings, flashing lights and humming machines.

When I awoke for the second time, I felt rather more lively, although unlikely to leap to my feet and perform complex dance steps. Luckily, this was not required of me and I settled for the more sedate raising of my arm to have my blood pressure taken once again. Satisfied noddings reassured me and I was informed that I would now return to the ward.

Anxiously, I looked around for the suited porter but he was nowhere to be seen. Instead, a tall, competent looking porter arrived and, accompanied by my usual entourage of nurses and clipboards, I sailed back into the ward, waving regally to my adoring public.

I was surprised by their looks of pure amazement. Had they not expected me to return or was there something rather unusual about my appearance? Later conversations elicited the fact that I had returned in such a short time that it was generally agreed that I could not possibly have had the operation already. The oxygen mask, drip and drainage tubes gave the lie to this theory and added to the confusion that was now erupting around me. It was with some difficulty that the assembled nurses hauled me across onto my bed, aided by the competent looking porter. I sank back into my pillows, closed my eyes once more and reviewed my situation. It was with considerable relief that I realised that I did not feel sick, I was not shuddering with cold and there was no pain to be felt anywhere.

Sleep beckoned me encouragingly and I obediently followed it into the pillowed depths.

I awoke a little later and smiled at the Hat who was watching me anxiously. Relieved, the Hat returned my smile and we conversed briefly on the state of my health. I confirmed that I was not feeling the cold at all. In fact, I was feeling extremely warm and rather uncomfortable but hesitated to complain as it seemed rather ungrateful given the obvious attempts that had been made to avoid my usual post-anaesthetic shudderings. A kindly nurse arrived to take my blood pressure and temperature and to offer me the ubiquitous cup of tea. I accepted with alacrity and a piece of my favourite cherry Genoa cake was added to the saucer along with the gentle advice to eat and drink slowly. I followed my instructions and then continued with my lively conversations in a way that belied my post-operative condition.

Time passed and the sun moved round until it was shining directly through the plate glass window and onto my already overheated body. A fan was found and placed in an appropriate position and the usual checks were performed. I was feeling extremely well and very glad to be alive. The oxygen mask was removed and at last, I discovered the reasons for my sweat-drenched skin. I reached under the bedclothes and found what appeared to be the end of a roll of cling-film. I pulled gently but the cling-film resisted, entrenching itself firmly into the creases of my stomach. I tugged once more but to no avail and the cling-film crowed triumphantly beneath the blankets. I changed tactics and took the cling-film by surprise while it was resting on its hard-won glory. With a sudden squelching sound, the cling-film gave up the struggle and concertinaed onto my surprised and bandaged chest. Winnie the Pooh and friends now lay soggily on my bedclothes in a tumbled heap as the cling-film revealed itself to be a special covering for warming up otherwise cold patients. I suspected that it was used in the children's ward to good effect but had escaped for a brief and relaxing break among adults. This particular adult was extremely grateful for its warming powers but felt no compunction at returning the blanket to a passing nurse and wishing Winnie and friends a fond, if slightly damp farewell.

The tea and cake were now sitting rather uncomfortably on my stomach and visiting times were looming. I decided it was time to make a quick trip to the loo. This entailed a lengthy trip through the rather small ward, out into the corridor and into the adjoining loo. I called a nurse who agreed to my request without hesitation as I seemed to be well on the way to recovery. The drip was unhooked by my willing acolyte and I was gently helped into a sitting position, albeit one still supported by pillows. The covers, now thankfully free of Winnie the Pooh, were lifted off my stockinged legs and tentatively, I swung them off the bed until they rested on the floor. There was still one more hurdle to be jumped before I would be ready to leap into action. Two long draining tubes were attached to the wound that lay hidden beneath the white dressings. These tubes led into a matching pair of bottles which were slowly filling with red-tinged liquid. In order to hide these rather unpleasant looking items and also to facilitate easier movement around the ward, each bottle had been placed in a cotton cover that would not have looked out of place in the accessory stores of the nineteen sixties. The violent op-art style patterns of swirling peach and pink were the perfect accessory for a first post-op outing. I reached back and hauled on the conveniently long handles. The acolyte then went round the other side of my bed and disentangled them from the bed wheels, threaded them through the legs of the table and deposited them in my hand.

Hesitantly, I slid towards the edge of the bed and came to an abrupt halt as the acolyte decided to choose that moment to remove the drip from my hand. I was free at last and slowly rose to a standing position. I would like to be able to say that I sailed out of the ward, carelessly swinging my matching bottle bags and waving a brief but confident au revoir to my companions. The truth was a little different. No sooner had I stood up than I sat down again fast. My head was spinning and I felt extremely sick and clammy. I was so close to fainting that I considered lying down again at once but didn't have the required energy for even that. The acolyte held me in a supporting sort of way and we considered our options. The need for the loo was growing a little more pressing and she suggested that a commode be brought in for me. It says something for my weakened state that I agreed without demur. However, when she returned wheeling a commode cunningly disguised as a wheelchair, we both agreed that as the ward was full of visitors that it might be more comfortable if I was wheeled out to the loo where essential activity would be more private.

In the end, I did sail out of the ward but it was not under my own steam if one can be pardoned a mix of metaphor. As we rounded the corner, I heard the Brother from the North enquiring after me and realised that he was standing near the desk accompanied by the parents and the Younger Daughter. This was not exactly the way I had planned to be following the operation but the acolyte had a good head of steam up now and ignoring my gathered family, we raced into the loo where she left me in peace. Some time later when I had finished throwing up, I decided it was time to summon the acolyte back to my side.

I have spent many hours in hospital wards as either patient or visitor and that long red cord has dangled before me, tempting me, causing me to panic in case I should inadvertently pull it instead of the light switch but never have I actually pulled it. My chance had come at last and I pulled enthusiastically. The acolyte returned and wheeled me back into the ward where my family stood ranged along the side of the bed. The Younger Daughter looked extremely anxious at the sight of me in a wheelchair, white lipped and trailing violently patterned bags behind me. Some considerable effort was deployed to return me to my bed and I sank gratefully back into my pillows. Sleep beckoned me after my exhausting outing and the family decanted to the café downstairs so that I could regain a little energy.

By the time they returned I had been sick once more and was feeling rather frail but tried to put on a brave face. The brave face decided that this was no place to be and tried to make a dash for freedom. I managed to restrain it for a few vital minutes until the family departed, reassured that I was at least alive if not exactly kicking. The brave face beat them to the door and disappeared down the corridor, leaving me to my own devices.

The next few minutes managed to combine elements of farce, panic and public humiliation. I mutely indicated that the rising nausea was unstoppable and a harassed nurse brought me a small grey cardboard bowl. Sadly the forces of nature were too powerful and the bowl proved inadequate to the task. It hung its head in shame as exclamations of horror mingled with pity rent the air. Its hours were numbered now and it carried its shame badly as it was consigned to a large plastic bin. The Hat looked on in great sympathy. She had undergone several chemo treatments and was a close acquaintance of sickness but even she could not understand the blind panic in my eyes. Nurses bustled round me with wordless mutterings and one of them finally thought to close the curtains thus reducing the level of humiliation a little.

Panic continued to mount in me but common sense was on the warpath and it fought a short but hard-won battle resulting in total victory as I realised that my pale yellow night shirt was not, in fact, now liberally covered with blood clots but half digested cherries from the cherry genoa cake. Panic retreated and I turned my attention to the next skirmish. It took two nurses to remove the offending night shirt, change the bed and re-clothe me in a delightful floral nightdress complete with lace trim and revolutionary back opening. This charming article of high fashion looked rather like a designer tent but at least it covered my rather large and flabby body which had so humiliatingly been revealed to the general public without even an x-rated certificate for company. The regret that I had only brought in one large T-shirt now made itself apparent and I determined to ask the Brother from the North to buy some more for me. Sleep called me once more and having submitted to the usual checks, consumed a small handful of tablets and firmly rejected the dinner of shepherd's pie which had been thoughtfully left on the table, I answered its insistent summons and slept.

Chapter Thirteen

The following day was hot and sunny and I felt rather like an ailing plant in a greenhouse. Nausea had decided that it would remain in place and was gaining in experience with every passing hour. After much discussion with nurses and doctors, I discovered that one of my painkillers contained codeine, a substance which I rarely take as it often makes me feel sick. Bureaucracy demanded permission from absent doctors before it could be withdrawn but in the meantime, a temporary solution was found by inserting a painkiller elsewhere in my poor battered body. My dignity peeped back round the cubicle curtains but decided that it needed a short break somewhere warm and sunny and disappeared with great speed.

A tray was placed on my table and I was ordered to eat my lunch. Hospital food has a **Reputation** with a capital R, in bold font and heavily underlined. I lifted the scratched metal lid covering the plate and viewed its contents with considerable misgiving. Identification was my first duty and that was proving extremely difficult. A small mound of some white substance lay congealing on the white plate. It was clothed in a glutinous white sauce which did nothing to aid recognition and plenty to encourage the flagging Nausea. A small branch of broccoli lay to one side, claiming to have been cooked 'al dente' but this would only be true if the 'dente' in question belonged to a particularly ferocious carnivore which spent much of its time sharpening its canines. I searched my memory in case the menu had imprinted itself on my mind but in vain. I had no idea what this could possibly be and decided to bring all my senses into play.

Sight had let me down and Taste was refusing to take part in the identification parade, aided and abetted in its decision by the ever mounting Nausea. Touch refused to be involved as it believed that its contribution would only add to existing humiliations by revealing to my usual audience a complete lack of manners. Hearing was not an option as the flaccid white mound on the plate remained resolutely silent. Thus it was left to Smell to come to my aid and it took on the task with enthusiasm but little success. A hesitant theory that fish might be involved somewhere was greeted with doubt but acceptance and I replaced the metal lid, turning my attention to the small plastic beaker that was also on the tray.

This seemed to contain an orange liquid and two or three objects that might just have been fruit. One of them closely resembled a cherry and Nausea returned to the fray fuelled by memories of the preceding day's events. Hospital food's **Reputation** was well deserved. I rejected the tray and decided that I needed a rest from decision making that would best be obtained by closing eyes and burying myself under the crisp clean sheets. Peace reigned.

Always an uneasy monarch, Peace was soon to face its greatest challenge in the person of a new addition to our little ward. She was outspoken, vociferous and loud of tone and she brought tension and irritation with her. She obviously knew a great deal about her illness and its treatment and did not hesitate to impart this information to everyone who came near her be they doctor, cleaner or other people's visitors. A visit to the loo or shower became a test of initiative as I had to pass her bed without making eye contact. The only respite came in the form of Rest Hour when doors were closed, footsteps quietened, televisions turned off and Peace returned to claim its throne for sixty short but most welcome minutes.

The ward slept.

When the doors opened to admit the usual rush of visitors, Pity entered as well as our newest neighbour deteriorated and became very obviously unwell. Reminded harshly of why we were all there, we became somewhat subdued until a nurse appeared at my bedside and announced brightly, "The Physio will be with you shortly." A shudder rippled around the ward. Covers were pulled up over noses and the occupants of the other beds slid out of sight.

The Physio! The image created by these words did not fit the young attractive blond who briskly entered the ward an hour or so later. Attired in a crisp clean white tunic that somehow managed to look sporty and efficient at the same time, she smiled gently. The smile belied the cruel streak that was later to emerge along with her true colours. A few questions later, surprisingly none of them concerning body-piercings, she handed me a frightening-looking leaflet which appeared to contain illustrated instructions for imitating land-based swimming. Gently, she stretched my left arm out in front of me. Gently, she raised it. Not so gently, she raised it higher. The Muscles and the Nerves surrounding the area recently vacated by the Young Leader complained, grumbling to each other. Pushed into action, they finally began to move. My arm was lowered and the incipient rebellion was halted in its tracks. Relief flooded through me but did not last long as seconds later, my arm was raised once more, higher this time.

The Muscles held a union meeting and decided that they would protest. Several of them contemplated a march comparable to the famous Jarrow march but maybe not quite so far. After all, it was very tiring being a Muscle and they needed to conserve their energy. The Nerves, meeting in a different area, sneered at the Muscles. They realised that they were getting the worst of this particular treatment and began to complain more vociferously and rather more painfully. The Crisp White Tunic listened to their complaints and obligingly lowered the arm again. I sank back against my pillows exhausted and the cruel streak emerged. Persuaded to sit up again, my arm was raised once more. The Muscles and the Nerves decided that it was time to join forces and stage a more efficient revolt. The Arm, looking down at them from its elevated position, felt nothing but pity for their futile complaints. It sympathised with them for they had gone through a great deal, but it remained confident that it would succeed in its quest as the Crisp White Tunic raised it even higher.

Lowered once more, the angle was now changed and the Arm was raised to the side. This woke up a different section of the Muscles and Nerves brigade. Sleepily, they rubbed their eyes, realising that the rumours were all true and battle was to be joined. The Arm, gracious in victory, moved up and down in a passable imitation of a wing and the Crisp White Tunic's gentle nature reasserted itself.

"I'll pop back later. Maybe we'll even be able to raise your arm to shoulder level then," she smiled. Shocked, the Muscles and the Nerves subsided. It was time to regroup.

"One last exercise!" The Crisp White Tunic smirked as she bent my right arm up behind my back and persuaded my reluctant left arm up and over my shoulder. As the fingers inched towards each other, the elbow reached up into the air and shouted aloud in triumph. The Muscles and the Nerves shouted aloud in painful protest but the fingers failed to touch.

The cruel streak decided to clock off for the day and left the gentle nature to return the arm to its normal position.

"Just four more times and that will do for today." The cruel streak seemed to have forgotten something and returned briefly for a little overtime. Gathering strength, the Arm performed the required manoeuvres. The Muscles and the Nerves found that their protest was wearing thin and one or two of them retreated, giving in gracefully. The Crisp White Tunic nudged the leaflet towards me.

"Practise a few times and I'll see you later," she said. Soft rubber soles left the ward and noses reappeared once more above the covers. Pity was in the eyes of all who looked on me. Practice could wait. Exercise was so exhausting and for now, sleep was beckoning and I responded willingly.

-

Chapter Fourteen

"I've come about the drains!"

I was startled into wakefulness by this comment and for a minute, I could not remember where I was. Had I contacted DynoRod for some reason? I was confused and disorientated but the question was repeated rather urgently by the harassed looking nurse bent over me.

"I've come to take one of them out," she said.

I mentally reassembled my senses which seemed to have taken off in different directions during my short doze and then nodded enthusiastically.

"Please do," I invited her.

Taking my drain out was not quite as simple as it sounded. Thankfully, the curtains had been drawn against the curious stares of my ward mates and somehow I could hear the unexpressed grumbles as they were deprived of some potentially lively entertainment. Following the incident with the rejected cherry genoa cake, my Brother from the North had braved the lingerie section of a well-known and reasonably cheap department store and he had purchased a selection of outsize night-shirts in various colours. One of these had replaced the voluminous and frilly hospital nightie and the sheep adorning its front complained as they were rolled up against their will. My will wasn't too happy either as the over-large stomach was now revealed, halted in the middle of its journey south. I rarely looked at my own body as the very sight of it had a tendency to inspire in me a feeling of nausea. Since Nausea already ruled my waking minutes, I did not feel that reinforcements were needed. The over-large stomach tried hard to make itself look small as it attempted to slide sideways but its days were numbered. Unaccustomed viewings of its pale slopes had reminded me of my pressing need to lose some weight and I took down a mental memo to do just that in the not too distant future.

The drain dressing was removed and an untangling of tubes ensued.

"This may feel rather strange," warned the harassed look and after a few seconds, she had my complete agreement. As the piece of transparent plastic tubing was slowly withdrawn, I felt as though it had been inserted as far as my toes. Why had they needed so much tubing? Why was it apparently coiled round my internal organs? What exactly had been draining away all this time? These questions and others in a similar vein were soon to be answered. Imagination had a great deal to answer for and it hung its head in shame as the truth was revealed and an extremely short length of tubing was finally pulled clear of my side. Surprise and relief battled for the position of prime emotion but relief won easily and was joined by comfort in its victory.

The tube's companion sulked, lying loosely on my exposed flesh. Some are chosen and some are not and the escaping tube sneered unpleasantly as it made its escape into a large green bag, accompanied by the disposable gloves, its attendant bottle and the garishly flowered bag that had held it for so long.

Dressings, nightshirt and dignity were replaced, curtains opened and I was informed that it was now rest hour as the harassed look departed the ward.

Rest hour was the best part of the day in the hospital routine. For one hour, everything came to a halt. Replete with lunch, patients sank back against their pillows. In my case today, lunch had consisted of a rather dry cracker and a piece of rubbery cheese as the unnamed fish in white sauce had somehow not seemed to tempt my appetite. My stomach, annoyed by all the attention being given to other parts of my body, had rebelled and for the first time in its life was turning down food. It will be obvious by now that I do not reject food lightly as I have a love affair with food that has lasted throughout my adult life. My senses had pulled rank over mere common sense and conspired to send me racing to fridge or larder far more frequently than was good for me. Lured onward by cheese, chocolate, mayonnaise and peanut butter, I had immersed myself in my passion and was now paying the price. Hospital food was doing everything in its meagre power to help common sense re-establish itself as the ruler of the other senses but the battle was hard. A brief stay in a private hospital for an eye operation had lulled my stomach into a false sense of security. There, I had eaten the most heavenly scrambled eggs I had ever tasted. Light, buttery and hot, they bore no resemblance to NHS scrambled eggs but even such delicious memories could not compensate for the food which lay before me and nausea was always on hand to reinforce the stomach's chosen course of action.

For now, dishes had been removed; headphones were plugged into televisions; telephones were diverted to the main desk; pillows were plumped and doors were closed. The busy life of the hospital was stilled and peace flooded in with the sunlight. It was a wonderful hour and one I wish I could repeat every day of my life. I would happily champion the cause of the more continental siesta as a vital addition to English lifestyle. No more noise or interruptions; no visitors allowed; no prodding or poking; no machines; no trolleys. Intrusions into this oasis of calm were only permitted in cases of emergency. At peace with my world and assured of a whole hour of enforced rest, I slept.

I woke in some confusion, surrounded by chatter and noise which jarred on my senses. I tried to open my eyes. The diagonally opposite patient with the loud and insistent voice, was being attended to by no less a personage than the manicurist. She filed and buffed and polished and they talked – not whispered but talked. As I was beginning to make sense of current events, I tried to focus my bleary eyes on my watch without much success. The manicurist moved across to the Hat opposite and continued her loud conversation. The Hat nodded apologetically in my direction and kept her replies to a whisper. Then the doors crashed open and a cleaner came in giving things a desultory wipe round with a cloth which looked as though it had seen better days and was ruing their disappearance. I realised that I must have slept for several hours but I could make sense of the figures on my watch. My eyelashes had taken advantage of the break in routine to become closely entwined with each other. Reluctantly, they said fond farewells, promising to write and meet again in the not too distant future as they began their painful separation. My eyes, released from their covering, glanced at ward clock and I realised with considerable annoyance that there was still half an hour of precious rest hour to go.

A pair of startled Eyebrows appeared at my bedside, attached to a cheery young man who looked no older than my teenage daughter but whose white coat and stethoscope proclaimed that he might just be a doctor. The crumpled shirt, buttoned incorrectly and the shadows under his eyes confirmed both my suspicions and his junior status.

"We think you might be able to go home today," he announced cheerfully. The Eyebrows seemed to be chasing after his receding hairline, giving him a look of permanent surprise which I assumed was not connected with the possibility of my going home.

Home. This is the word which every hospital patient longs to hear and the problems incurred by the day to day running of the home and demands of family and friends vanished from memory as the prospect of going home took hold.

I reviewed my situation and I wasn't only the one. The superbugs lurking unseen in every corner of the ward reviewed the situation as well. They had been waiting to make their attack as they assembled in corners unreached by mops, dusters or hoovers and they conferred soundlessly. Would this patient escape their planned attack? Should she really be allowed to leave without their calling card attached? My own considerations did not involve superbugs of any variety. Nausea was still a close companion although its influence was fading with every hour following the withdrawal of my painkillers and I was a little unsteady on my legs. One reluctant drain remained in place and I did not want to take the tube home with me as we were not on speaking terms, each of us wishing that he could be removed. He pulled and tugged at my dressings and wound himself round the edge of the bed when I wanted to get up, bringing me up short and painfully. To add to the problems, the flowery bag spent much of its time formulating an escape plan in an attempt to rejoin its departed twin. I decided that I would prefer to remain in hospital until the planned departure day of Thursday – just one more day.

When I announced my decision, the fugitive

Eyebrows tried to reassert themselves as a puzzled frown but this attempt was doomed to disappointment and as I explained my reasons, they conceded defeat. They continued their race towards the hairline as the junior doctor reassured me that my decision was acceptable. By Thursday, I would have parted company with my drain and would be able to return home unencumbered by its sulky presence. The superbugs cheered silently not realising that in this hospital, their success levels were limited and that one more patient would soon be escaping from their clutches.

The afternoon stretched ahead of me. A time to be filled with laughter and light conversation, catching up with the activities of the Younger Daughter and the Brother from the North and culminating in the successful consumption of cottage pie and broccoli. As night drew closer and the lights were dimmed, I began to turn my thoughts to home and all that lay ahead of me.

Home beckoned me but various hurdles would have to be jumped and jumping was the last thing on my mind that night as I lay tucked into newly laundered sheets, fresh water at my side and the knowledge that someone else would be cooking and washing up for me for a few more precious hours. The Brother from the North would be able to stay for a day or so longer and the freezer was stocked with food. Throughout my temporary absence, meals had been arriving on the doorstep, courtesy of the members of my women's Bible study group at church. Pasta bakes, chicken casseroles, curries and stews arrived in quick succession accompanied by rice dishes, salads and potatoes in a variety of guises. The Younger Daughter possessed a small and selective appetite and had been provided with her very own individual portions of her favourite shepherd's pie. In vain did the Brother from the North protest that he was a very good cook himself and more than competent to provide meals for the two of them. The dishes kept on arriving as my dear friends desperately found a way of supporting me. A rota was pinned to the notice board in the hall and I recalled that it would cover the first few days of my arrival home as well. Food would not be a problem.

The Easter holidays were due to start the day after my release and the Younger Daughter would provide me with companionship and assistance where necessary. She would be joined, albeit briefly, by the Older Daughter and a succession of willing friends and neighbours. I would not have to lift a finger. Peace of Mind entered the ward and crept into bed with me, stilling my anxieties and closing my eyelids. Obediently, I abandoned myself to sleep and my last night in the Hospital.

Chapter Fifteen

The night had been filled with hurrying footsteps, urgent whispers, stifled weeping and once, the creaking wheels of the mortuary trolley as it carried its sad burden away from the ward. All had not been peace and quiet in my own small section of the ward and I was often woken by the rattling of curtain rings as yet another white-coated shape slipped into the cubicle diagonally opposite me. More whisperings accompanied other, harsher sounds and lights flicked on and off as bells summoned various nurses. In the middle of the night, my sense of humour decided that it needed some respite and took to its heels, abandoning me to the harsh realities of life on a cancer ward. I buried my head in the metaphorical sand represented by my pillow and tried to sleep but my dreams were of twisted tubes, badly-lit tunnels and pale, eerie shapes set against a background of pulsing lights and disembodied screams. I was glad when I finally awoke to a misty grey dawn – a dawn which could be my last in the Hospital.

A weary-looking nurse arrived at my bedside pushing her trolley before her. Her black-shadowed eyes revealed the horrors of the night and she worked hastily in order to get all paperwork completed before the hand-over and her release into the outside world. My arm was wrapped in the wide blood pressure cuff, a thermometer was plunged into my ear and a pen was gripped between her teeth as she fought with papers and machines. The pen flicked upwards in astonishment as numbers flickered into life on the machine beside me. I soon shared in the astonishment as the figures were entered onto my chart. It seemed that the weary-looking nurse had no energy left for bewilderment and she read out her findings in a flat, unsurprised voice.

"Pulse is 37."

I pinched myself. With a pulse of 37, I figured I was quite possibly in some sort of suspended animation, a feeling which was compounded by her next remark, "Temperature is 73 degrees celsius."

Maybe suspended animation was too lively a condition for someone with such a high temperature but I fought my way back to life with a mild suggestion that there might be some mistake. The weary-looking nurse shook herself out of her inertia and entered the correct temperature (37) and pulse (73). She assured me that my blood pressure was stable and went off down the ward laughing to herself. I was glad to have been responsible for bringing a little light relief to her otherwise ghastly shift.

I turned my attention to the welcome arrival of tea and toast which were consumed in silence in deference to the early hour and cold grey light filtering in through the blinds. My sense of humour which had been lurking somewhere outside the ward, decided that it was safe to return and I welcomed it back with enthusiasm. The Hat nodded at me encouragingly and soon we were deep in conversation, joined by the two senses of humour and the occasional passing nurse.

Reassured by one such nurse that the bathroom was free, I began to prepare for my daily ablutions. This was made rather difficult by the activities of my remaining drain tube. I do not know if it was the shock caused by my rogue readings or the fact that the breakfast toast had been hot, but my tube had tried to hide under the bed. It had become inextricably linked with the wheels of my bedside table and was discovering a very close affinity to my slippers. Meanwhile, the bottle, in its jaunty cover, had wound itself round the arm of the chair and was hanging upside down in a rather alarming manner.

My attempts to free the tube provided several minutes of entertainment for the Hat and very nearly necessitated a visit to the fracture clinic but I persevered and finally raised the bottle high above my head in celebration. All inhabitants of the ward were extremely grateful that the wildly coloured bag remained in place, concealing the contents of the bottle from their somewhat startled gaze. Common Sense reasserted itself and I busied myself in attempting to locate slippers, towel and wash bag. Red-faced from my exertions but triumphant, I laid out my trophies on the bed , disentangled the tube once more and had just put on my slippers when a badge appeared at my side, firmly attached to its owner, proudly proclaiming her to be a 'clinical nurse specialist'. The badge invited me to accompany her to her office just along the ward and to bring a bra. I hesitated for a brief moment while vanity fought with the need for speed but there were no mirrors on the ward and vanity lost the battle.

I rose from my bed and meekly followed the badge out of my cosy four-bedded room and down the corridor. Vanity shrugged and washed its hands of me. I must have been an attractive sight. I am not known for the smallness of my physique, being in fact, extremely overweight and large busted (on one side at least). I had not washed my short spiky hair for two days and although one side of the hair was lying submissively against my head, the other side was doing a passable audition for Woody Woodpecker, being both red and erect. The over large T-shirt that I wore as a nightie did not reach down as far as the long white surgical support stockings which, in turn, were attached to grey felt slippers. As I neared the end of the ward, I began to panic and held back a little. Briskly encouraged by the two nurses ahead of me, I dutifully passed through the double doors and out into the corridor. There were people out here! People who were not patients or nurses from my ward and I felt extremely vulnerable. I was absolutely certain that everyone was staring at me with barely concealed horror. Much later, I realised that in a specialist cancer hospital, everyone is too consumed by their own problems to be aware of anyone else but it was with some relief that I rounded a corner and entered a small office. Safe at last!

The Badge gestured to a seat and proceeded to initiate me in the secrets of the 'comfie'. This is a soft cloth cover apparently filled with toy stuffing which is slipped inside the bra to act as a surrogate breast until the day comes for the fitting of the prosthesis. Safely concealed beneath my voluminous t-shirt, E-Cup sneered at the flattish 'comfie' that was produced for my inspection. With the eye of an expert, the Badge swiftly sized me up and went in search of the bag of toy stuffing. She proceeded to ram into the 'comfie' as much of the stuffing as she was able before holding up the resultant lumpy bag for my considered inspection. The interview then descended into the realms of horror films as the Badge bade me remove my t-shirt and look into the full-length mirror. I am not on good terms with the whole concept of full-length mirrors and avoid them wherever possible. Department store changing rooms with mirrors that can simultaneously reveal the horrors of front and rear have been known to reduce me to a sobbing and hysterical wreck. Mirrors in my house are used solely for checking the latest hair -style, the accuracy of lipstick application and the presence of spinach between my teeth. Never will I willingly stand before such a mirror and gaze upon my person. Certainly, I would not choose to do so clad in grey felt slippers, long white surgical stockings, over-large knickers , a large taped dressing pad covering the absence of the once loved C-cup and the ubiquitous drain tube with its attached bottle in multicoloured bag.

I gritted my teeth, summoned my sense of humour from where it was hiding outside the door and gazed at my reflection. E-cup hung its head down low and was joined in its perusal of the floor by my deeply ashamed stomach. My hair tried standing up proudly but failed dismally and the whole attention of my being centred on the gash of white bandaging across my chest. The sense of humour rallied to the occasion and I made a few amusing comments to the Badge who was watching me anxiously. Then the bra that had dangled from my fingers was gently fastened round my chest and the 'comfie' inserted into the puckered and empty left cup. The stuffing was tweaked and more added to balance the two sides. I put on the huge purple T-shirt and gazed back at my reflection. Normality seemed to have been restored and I relaxed a little before giving up my new shape to the Badge. She helped me out of my bra once again and placed the somewhat lumpy 'comfie' in a plastic bag with extra handfuls of toy stuffing, presumably in case E-cup expanded to a size 'F' and balance was needed. Hastily, I replaced my t-shirt and left her small domain armed with two 'comfies' (one on and one in the wash), a large tub of aqueous cream, the telephone number of the prosthesis clinic and three catalogues devoted entirely to mastectomy wear. Clutching my booty, I took my humiliated and still unwashed body back to the ward to be rewarded by a cup of tea and a ginger biscuit.

Minutes later, a nurse appeared at my bedside to remove the drain. I was an old hand at this procedure by now and barely flinched although its removal was not without discomfort. I bade a fond farewell to the swirling patterns of the bag and finally made it into the bathroom for a much needed wash. Thus it was that I was at least clean when the junior doctor appeared with my release forms and the promise that my return home was now confirmed.

A phone call was made to the waiting Brother from the North, my bag was packed and I was given packs of replacement dressings and tape. Forms were signed, appointments given for six months hence, farewells and thank yous said and then I gingerly made my way out into the chilly car park. I cannot recommend the wearing of a seat belt when one has had such radical breast surgery but the 'comfie' finally came into its own from its position hidden inside my bra. Triumphantly, it announced its protection of me from the pressure of the belt and E-cup acknowledged a temporary truce as we made our way back home.

<u>Chapter Sixteen</u>

Home was all I remembered it to be, a place of calm, of warmth, of palatable food and comfort and once ensconced on my sofa, I did the only logical thing and fell fast asleep. When I awoke some time later, the Younger Daughter was home from school, a cup of tea stood steaming gently beside me and the Brother from the North was clutching handfuls of envelopes. In all, I received eighty four cards so full of love, support, prayer and encouragement that I was often reduced to unexpected tears. Every available surface was now covered with pictures of flowers, cats and arty prints and I realised that dusting would be out of the question for some time. There seems to be no law governing the length of time that cards should be kept on display and I reasoned that eight months seemed as good a time scale as any. This would bring me to December when the Get Well cards could be replaced by Christmas cards and the dusting avoided for a further month or so.

My cogitations were interrupted by the arrival of a huge urn filled with plants, a gift from my wonderful Bible Study group. These women had prayed for me, provided meals for the Brother from the North, the Younger Daughter and now me and had clubbed together to buy me something so beautiful that it still delights me every time I look out at my patio. The accompanying card was filled with yet more loving greetings, including one from a member who was fighting her own battle with cancer. Sadly, she was to lose her battle later in the year and it was only after her funeral that I realised that she had, long ago, been a close friend and flatmate of the Brother from the North. It is a small world we inhabit.

It was wonderful to be back in my own bed, without the constant interruptions and strange noises that are part of hospital life. I took advantage of the peace and slept well, free of drains and surgical stockings. The morning would bring its own challenges.

I needed to wash the smell of hospitals away from my skin and hair and decided that a shower must take priority over any other activity. In order to keep the dressing dry, I taped a plastic bag over it and then assumed a Yogic stance in the bath. My body was contorted into unnatural positions as I attempted to wash my hair and shower without actually getting water onto my chest. The water had other ideas and slid unnoticed over my shoulders, insinuating itself down what had once been a substantial cleavage and now rather resembled an undulating escarpment with a sharp drop. However, the plastic bag resisted valiantly and the dressing remained dry. Exhausted by my efforts, I retired to the sofa once more and dozed pleasantly until the arrival of the first of many visitors that day.

The following day saw the arrival of the Older Daughter from a school trip from France to Ireland. She was en route to a week's work in a bookshop at a

Christian Festival and stayed only long enough to reassure herself that I was doing as well as could be expected and to do her washing. She departed for Lincolnshire and shortly afterwards, I said a sad farewell to the wonderful Brother from the North. I owed him so much and knew he was returning to his own problems, put on hold while he cared for us. The Younger Daughter, the Parents and the Friends leapt into the breach and I was never short of company or food!

Days passed and I grew stronger and more able to take up the reins of the household once again. I attempted to have a bath and quickly discovered that the only way I could lever my body out of the water was to turn onto my stomach like a beached whale and manoeuvre myself onto my knees before rising to my unsteady feet and clambering out of the bath. It was to be over a year before I was able to push up on my arm and leave the bath in a less undignified manner.

Meanwhile, the outside world beckoned and I attempted to put on my socks. As has been seen, this was not an entirely successful venture and failure smirked as I retired once more to my sofa. However, failure's victory was short-lived and a day later, I successfully managed the short walk to the post box. On Easter Sunday, I even managed to get to church and was overwhelmed by the warmth of my welcome back. Hugs were given rather too enthusiastically at times and all my latent acting skills were summoned as I accepted them without flinching. The emotional pleasure more than compensated for the physical pain and I happily returned the hugs.

Six weeks later, I was once more allowed to drive and my first outing was, of course, a return trip to the Hospital. I had made an appointment for a consultation at the Prosthetics Clinic and duly made my way to the upper reaches of the Hospital. Tucked securely into my bag was my new bra. This bra was the size of a small hammock and conveniently possessed a pocket in both sides. I considered the tiny slit cut into each pocket and reasoned that the prosthesis must be small and very flexible. Flooded with relief, I reached the unassuming room marked 'Prosthetics' and entered my new world.

I was greeted by a tired smile that seemed to have seen everything that day and had no energy for any more problems. I explained my mission and was asked to remove my upper garments and hold my arms above my head. This was no mean feat in spite of daily physiotherapy and my right arm smirked unpleasantly as it shot into the air and remained clamped to my ear, straight and pointed directly towards the ceiling. Apologetically, my left arm raised itself as far as possible and pointed directly towards the weary smile. The smile gathered its manners and managed to wind the tape measure around my chest. I pondered my remaining E- cup and wondered what measurement would result from my new asymmetric shape.

The smile faded as it informed me that I was quite large, a fact I already knew to my shame, and instructed me to sit and wait. I shivered in the silence of the cool room and waited. The smile returned but was now hidden behind a pile of what looked like huge shoe boxes. When it reappeared, it had been replaced by a look of weary resignation, the change obviously prompted by experience as the pile of boxes hit the ground and we started the long process of attempting to find a suitable (and large) prosthesis. The pockets in the bra cowered in fear and feelings of inadequacy.

The first prosthesis was removed from its box where it lay nestled in a plastic container moulded to its own size and shape. E-cup gasped in amazement as the massive silicon Shape appeared, apparently moving of its own accord and spilling over its supporting hand. The smile briefly reappeared but soon vanished as the Battle of the Pocket began. The Shape was twisted, folded and squeezed but the brave little pocket resisted all attempts to breach its confines. The Battle was long and frustrating and it is to the pocket's credit that it only surrendered when confronted by the threat of a huge pair of scissors. At last, the Shape was forced into the pocket and I was allowed to stand once more to be fitted with this monstrosity. The bra was done up firmly and the Shape forced into the correct position. I was then asked to pose in front of the mirror, not my favourite activity at the best of times, and stare hard at my new figure. An enormous shelf seemed to have landed on my body and E-cup had shrunk into insignificance. "Too big" came the verdict and the whole procedure was first reversed and then attempted with a slightly smaller shape. The pocket had conceded defeat and so the Battle was more of a minor skirmish this time.

By the time the fourth shape was being considered by us all, I had developed sympathy for the vanished smile and my own sense of humour had gone for a long walk in the scrubland opposite the Hospital. However, this was announced to be a success and the proud and successful Shape was removed to its nest once more, secure in the knowledge that it had found a new home at last. I resumed the wearing of my small and soft 'comfie' and carried my huge box back to the car, leaving the now exhausted smile to collect the boxes and return them to their shelves to await a more enthusiastic reception from another client.

Once home, I opened my box and read the care instructions with growing dismay and considered getting a puppy instead as it would need less care than this amorphous blob of silicon. I started my new regime the next morning and quickly realised that I would have to get up a lot earlier if I wished to leave the house on time.

It took twenty minutes to force the Shape into the resisting little pocket and another five to attempt to do up my bra behind my back while the heavy front pulled hard in the opposite direction. My sense of humour had still not returned from its travels and indeed would take a well-earned break for a few days as I got to grips with my new companion. By bedtime, I was eagerly looking forward to removing this extra weight from my chest but the night time routine involved another fight with the now over-stretched pocket, a gentle bath in tepid water (for the Shape, not me), the use of a soft towel to pat it dry and then the careful placing of the Shape reverently in its plastic nest where it would rest for the night. I fell into bed exhausted and tense, waking the next day unrefreshed and quite unprepared for yet another battle. Time did not make this procedure any easier and I found that anger was quickly replacing the absent sense of humour. In addition to the anger, my neck had decided that it needed attention too and quickly developed a combination of sharp pains and dull aches that led to a constant headache.

Meanwhile, I had returned to school and there I discovered yet another problem. Infant children are short in stature and generally sit on rather small chairs as do their teachers. Herein lay my new difficulty. I often had to kneel down beside a child to hear it read, do up a shoelace, listen to whispered complaints or help with the challenge of holding a pencil. This had been my custom for many years, but now when I knelt down, I also tipped forward landing head first on the floor much to the surprise of the infant beside me. Several of them got into the habit of crouching at my head to continue their whisperings rather than assist me to my knees again. This caused several raised eyebrows when parents were being shown round the school and I soon realised that something would have to be done to rectify the situation. The scenario was repeated at home when bending to pick something up off the floor, trying to put washing into the machine or stroking the cat. This was no way to live and the headache and the neck called a meeting with the balance mechanisms to decide on a new course of action.

Chapter Seventeen

The next few days saw a flurry of activity as I sought an acceptable answer to my problems. An Idea took root and began to grow, spreading its tentacles through my somewhat confused brain in an attempt to bring relief to my neck, my back and my dignity. In my search for freedom from pain, I engaged my favourite companion – my trusty computer and its easy access to the world in the form of the internet. I typed the Idea into Google and sat back hopefully. Many offerings spread themselves across the screen offering breast reconstructions, foam filled prostheses (the 'comfie' smirked from its position in my underwear drawer) and catalogues displaying an alarming variety of swimming costumes and outsized bras. Hidden amongst these delights lay one little website that offered me hope and I clicked on it with enthusiasm. It belonged to two Dutch women who had opted not to wear their prostheses and had designed clothing that would act as a distraction to the eye. These were not women who were out to make money from selling wildly expensive designer clothing, but rather two friends who wanted to share their skills in clothing adaptation.

With growing enthusiasm, I perused the pictures

and the Idea preened itself rather smugly as it sensed the anguish that was being experienced by the Silicon Blob whose days now seemed numbered. I managed to make it upstairs without being pulled forward onto each step and began to empty the contents of drawers and cupboards into my bed. Some time later, I approached the room belonging to the Older Daughter and knocked gently on the door. Suddenly the Idea had taken fright and had waited behind in my room, peering out from behind the enthusiasm that had carried me thus far. The Silicon Blob lay abandoned on the bed, all but covered with a heap of vest tops and scarves. The Older Daughter opened the door and confidence came back to help me as I twirled and posed before her.

"What do you think?" I asked, and my confidence began to shrink slightly before her puzzled gaze. Puzzlement spread from her eyes to her voice as she said,

"Er...very nice but what am I looking at? What's new?"

I was wearing a black vest top and a thin pink shirt with a large hair clip in the shape of a black flower firmly clipped to its left hand lapel. I had found the hair clip in a small drawer full of odds and ends which includes my passport, some safety pins, a tube of glue, the red book containing the birth records of both children, a compass and a number of hair clips among other things. I have no idea why the hair clips were there as I have had very short hair for many years but they seemed to be the answer to my quest.

I confess to be slightly disappointed by the unenthusiastic response of the Older Daughter and so dragged the Younger Daughter into the discussion. However, she too, seemed to be unimpressed as I did not look significantly different from usual – apart from the large flower on my shirt. Back in my room, the Idea cheered silently and then I realised that it was a resounding success. The flower had done its job and distracted the mind from the flatness beneath it. When the Daughters realised the function of the flower, they became excited and enthusiastic in their support and the next hour was spent in a whirl of scarves and more flowery clips as I searched for combinations of clothes that would disguise the lack of C-cup and its poor replacement, the Silicon Blob.

The next day, I braved an excursion into my local town leaving the Blob at home, hiding its shame in its nest. I felt acutely aware of my lopsided shape and the occasional puzzled glance, but few people will risk staring at that area of any woman's body in case accusations of improper behaviour come their way. On my travels through the town, I noticed a woman with only one leg making her way slowly through the crowds. A few people glanced sympathetically at her and some risked a second glance, but no-one challenged her or questioned her decision not to wear an artificial leg and I gained confidence from our similarity. School would prove to be a slightly different challenge as Infants are notoriously frank in their observations. One beautiful sunny day, I was brought up short while doing playground duty when three little girls approached me and accused me of only having one 'booby' and wanting to know the reason why. I replied that there had been something wrong with the other one but that I was absolutely fine now.

One little girl ran off refusing to speak to me anymore. One of the remaining two reassured me that she loved me no matter what I looked like. She continued that she had noticed some time ago but that she had thought it rather rude to mention it to me.

I was then escorted lovingly up the steps and back to class where I was watched over protectively for the rest of the day. The third little girl thought she might be able to speak to me again one day and indeed, the following day, she was chatting to me in her usual way.

Only one other person has ever made a negative comment to me and she leaned across a counter at church where I was serving coffee and accused me of being a disgrace to femininity. I was rather taken aback but decided that the problem lay with her and not with me, a tenet I have clung to ever since. Several people have tried to convince me that the Blob was a good idea and that I should try again. These included doctors, nurses, bra fitters at my local department store and the mastectomy specialist at the hospital but I remained determined in my chosen route and do so to this very day. The Silicon Blob was later confined to a box in the loft out of my sight and thence to the local corporation dump where its humiliation and shame were buried amongst the other abandoned detritus of human living. The Idea was triumphant in its success and was awarded a medal by the neck and the back as pain receded from them. Balance was restored and I stopped keeling over every time I leant forwards. An additional benefit came in the realisation that I was no longer being made daily aware of my skirmish with cancer. The Blob had felt like an alien pressed against my chest. Without it, my chest feels normal and it is only when I look in the mirror that I remember. However, now I can look at it all with gratitude for yet another escape thanks to medical science and my own perseverance, my faith and my amazing family and friends.

Post Script

Nearly ten years have passed much to my amazement and whilst they have not been uneventful, I remain positive and well. There have been scares along the way which necessitated more bone scans but all were clear. A perforated, gangrenous appendix made a surprise incursion into my life and added another battle scar to my poor body but surprisingly the scariest words I heard were, "You are now fully discharged from this hospital and no longer need annual mammograms and appointments.

These words filled me with panic and anxiety as I had been a regular attender at that specialist hospital for nearly twenty five years but now I live with the normality experienced by most women.

People have moved on and away and the Great Italian succumbed to his own hidden illness but others carry on his work and I offer thanks to them and the researchers who have been responsible for saving so many lives as well as all those amazing people who supported me along the way and continue to do so every day.

Lynne Mattick

ABOUT THE AUTHOR

Lynne Mattick trained as a French teacher and is currently teaching in an infant school. She spent four years at Teacher Training College near Manchester and a year in France but now lives near London with one of her daughters and her cat. She has always dreamed of becoming a writer. Maybe her dreams are coming true as she approaches retirement.

7483905R00067

Printed in Great Britain
by Amazon.co.uk, Ltd.,
Marston Gate.